Multicultural Health Care and Rehabilitation of Older People

Edited by

Amanda Squires

Edward Arnold
A division of Hodder & Stoughton
LONDON MELBOURNE AUCKLAND

© 1991 Amanda J. Squires

First published in Great Britain 1991

British Library Cataloguing in Publication Data
Squires, Amanda J.
  Multicultural health care and rehabilitation of older people
  I. Title
362.6089

ISBN 0-340-54362-0

Typeset in 10/11 pt Ehrhardt by Hewer Text Composition Services, Edinburgh
Printed and bound in Great Britain for Edward Arnold,
a division of Hodder and Stoughton Limited, Mill Road,
Dunton Green, Sevenoaks, Kent TN13 2YA by
Biddles Limited, Guildford and King's Lynn

Contents

In this section, specialists look at their role, identifying and examining the salient issues in their particular fields.

Contributors

Alison Blenkinsop B.Pharm, PhD, MRPharmS, Pharmacy Practice Fellow, University of Bradford

Charon Bansal MChS, SRCh, Senior Chiropodist, Newham Health Authority

Deirdre Duncan PhD, MSc, Dip CST, MCST, Senior Lecturer, School of Speech Therapy, Birmingham Polytechnic

Steve Fenton PhD, MA, Senior Lecturer in Sociology, University of Bristol; Co-Director, Centre for the Study of Minorities and Social Change

James George MB, ChB, MRCP, Consultant Physician in Geriatric Medicine, Cumberland Infirmary, Carlisle

Margaret Heatley BSc, MCSP, SRP, Superintendent Physiotherapist, Tower Hamlets Health Authority, London

Clephane Hume BA, DipCOT, SROT, Lecturer, Queen Margaret College, Edinburgh

Bernard Lau MB, BS (HK), MRCPsych (UK), DPM (RCP.Lond. RCS.Eng), Consultant Psychiatrist, St Paul's Hospital, Hong Kong

Paul McKeigue MA, MSc, MB, BChir, MFCM, Senior Lecturer, Department of Epidemiology and Population Sciences, London School of Hygiene and Tropical Medicine

Simeon Onyejiako Ll.B.

Seema Padihar MChs, D Pod M, SRCh, District Chiropody Manager, Newham Health Authority

Rhona Panton MPhil, MRPharmS, Regional Pharmaceutical Officer, West Midlands Regional Health Authority

Indoo Partop BA, *formerly* Researcher on Ethnic Minorities and Pharmacy, Aston University

Shushila Patel BA, Senior Equal Opportunities Advisor, Tower Hamlets Health Authority

Ruth Prime BA, Social Services Inspector, Department of Health, London

Bashir Qureshi FRCGP, DCH, AFOM(RCP), FRSH, MICGP, FRIPHH, General Practitioner and Community Health Officer, Hounslow, Middlesex

Pam Schweitzer BA, Artistic Director, Age Exchange Theatre Trust, London

Kiran Shukla BSc, BEd, SRD, District Dietitian, Basildon and Thurrock Health Authority

Amanda Squires MSc, Grad Dip Phys, MCSP, SRP, Formerly District
Physiotherapist, Waltham Forest Health Authority

Liz Stewart Dip. Guid.&Couns Personnel Manager, (Equal Opportunities)
Advisor, Waltham Forest Health Authority

Arlene Trim BSc (Hons), RGN, SCM. RSCN, HV, Senior Lecturer in Health
Studies, Croydon College

Durreshahwar Wassim Co-ordinator, Asian Elderly Concern, Walthamstow,
London.

John Young MB, Bs(Hons), MSC, MRCP, Consultant Geriatrician, Bradford

Acknowledgements

The authors wish to thank all the patients, clients and colleagues who have wittingly and unwittingly contributed to this book, and in particular Mrs A. Martin for preparing the manuscript for Chapter 2, and P. Fenn Clark and G. Revell for helpful comments on the manuscript for Chapter 12. Particular acknowledgement is given to the Librarians of The Kings Fund The Centre of Policy on Ageing and Age Concern England. Also to the Standing Committee for Ethnic Minority Elders for advice at the conceptual stage of the book, and to Vertec Scientific Ltd. for information on bone density.

Foreword

Ageing of ethnic minority groups in Britain is occurring rapidly, and is beginning to be noticed by health and social services staff in most of the large cities and towns in Britain. Many of us now have black and Asian elderly patients on our wards or practice lists, and in our day hospitals and centres. The response of health and social services has typically been defined in terms of 'the problems' of black and Asian people, further stigmatising them, and ignoring those ethnic minorities who are not readily distinguishable by their skin colour. The problems reside with the jeopardies that face ethnic elders: those of age, of racism, of limited access to services, of poverty, and not necessarily with a lack of English, different customs and beliefs, or 'exotic' illnesses.

There is a feeling that we should be doing a better job for our ethnic minority patients, in particular that we need more interpreters and more training in appropriate languages for communication with patients, and more training for staff. Implementation of the NHS and Community Care Act of 1990 is likely to increase awareness of the need for health services to serve local (including ethnic minority) community needs. These are only partial solutions to the jeopardies faced by ethnic elders.

Although there is a wealth of literature about ethnic minorities there has been remarkably little systematic study of the impact of ageing – on the psyche, on social networks, and on physical health, and virtually no research making comparisons with the experience of the host community. This lack of information has not deterred the contributors to this book who have adopted various strategies in writing about the responses they as professionals make to ethnic elders. The service principles (such as good communication and teamwork, respect for the patient) that work for the indigenous patient should work for the others also. Several authors have used case examples to highlight good practice. An imaginative alternative is to define the concerns, hopes and dreams of ethnic minorities using reminiscence and theatre; Schweitzer's chapter deserves to be widely read, and should sweep aside a number of myths and stereotypes.

Little is said about disability and handicap, or the patterns of disease amongst ethnic elders, largely because there has been little systematic study. Instead much is made of the transitional nature of ethnic minorities; the extent to which ethnic elders cling onto home culture or assimilate the new host culture. It is unlikely that any simple formula applies to this complex aspect of life. Readers will discover many prejudices and stereotypes described throughout the book – and in identifying these may be able better to recognise their own.

This book is a necessary first step in laying out some of the issues. It is ambitious in its scope, and in its desire to point the way forward. Some policies and practices revealed in this book will infuriate, some will educate, some will confuse and contradict. But that is the nature of this topic; we have too little information and know too little about the impact of what we as practitioners do for ethnic minorities to see the way forward with any clarity. As ethnic minorities age, experience will grow and a firm foundation for a specific rehabilitation approach for ethnic elders will be established.

Shah Ebrahim
Professor of Health Care of the Elderly
The London Hospital Medical College and St. Bartholomew's Hospital Medical College, London
1991

Introduction

At the inception of the NHS in 1948, staff were to treat all patients irrespective of race, religion or creed. The Race Relations Act of 1976 acknowledged that Britain had become a multicultural society. The NHS and Community Care Act (1990) not only requires the needs of the population to be identified, but emphasises that 'people from different cultural background may have particular care needs and problems'. This book brings together, for the first time, the relevance of a multicultural society to the multidisciplinary provision of health and social services by describing the cultural, social and health aspects that need to be applied to unique populations. The recognition that attitudes and expectations differ is a key theme and a diversity of views have been sought.

The immigration to Britain (mainly since the 1930) of economically active people from other countries for political and economic reasons, has meant that for the first time in the history of the care of older people, significant numbers of ethnic minority elders are, and will be, needing health care and social services. In some parts of Britain, where ethnic minority communities already exist, knowledge is beginning to be acquired on which to plan and provide services.

Transcultural medicine has been described as the knowledge of medical and communication encounters between health workers and patients of different ethnic groups, and this book aims to assist in the understanding of these communication needs which also extend to the relationships between members of the health team itself.

The health and social needs of this section of the population may have some similarities with the indigenous population, but there may be differences in presentation of disease, its significance, and both physical and psychological response to treatment. Access to services may also differ and these issues need to be understood and addressed as effective care must be acceptable care. Mental illness is not covered in depth but noted as an essential issue in holistic care and alert readers to its likely existance in minority groups as a response to the stress experienced.

The social needs of ethnic elders are also complex, particularly in view of the three-generation traditional family structure, the Western upbringing and consequent attitudes of the children and grandchildren of elders, and in particular the duration of contact with the British culture. Isolation and loneliness are often underestimated. Housing and employment of people from ethnic minorities also has considerable repercussions for older people due to benefit entitlement and particular housing requirements for disabilities.

The position of the ethnic minority formal carer in this system is invidious. There is an expectation of a style of work within a system designed largely by and for the majority population, at the same time considering the needs of the relatives, the patient and his or her colleagues, as well as their own personal beliefs about health and social care.

This book is intended as a first point of reference for care staff, planners and educators. The history of immigration to Britain of a variety of groups supplies a context for developing health trends, traditional beliefs, medical needs and the use of both traditional and Western medicine. Contributors from a variety of specialist backgrounds demonstrate how perceived difficulties can be overcome, show examples of good practice, and make suggestions for future planning. As with most challenges, understanding of the issues, working with colleagues to share knowledge and experience, education at all levels, and above all seeking information from the client group, are the key points to apply within an identified population.

This book has been produced for the British system with its unique cultural mix and social history, but much can be applied to similar situations elsewhere where countries have been, by tradition, recipients of multicultural migration. The book does not aim to solve all the problems but rather to raise awareness of the issues and encourage readers to seek further information once it is accepted that a change in traditional attitudes is needed.

Amanda Squires

Section I Ethnic Minorities in the United Kingdom

This section examines the history and background of minority groups in Britain to set a context for issues discussed later, and identifies areas for special consideration.

1

Ethnic minority populations in the United Kingdom

Steve Fenton

British society

In the making of British society there have been many and various influences on the development of the population – Roman, Scandinavian, French – including invasion, conquest and migration. Britain has never been an 'immigrant receiving society' on the scale of the United States. In, for example, Chicago in 1890 some 41 per cent of the population was foreign-born; no British city will have had such a proportion born outside the country. The 1981 Census revealed Greater London's foreign-born population to be about 18 per cent of the total; those born outside the United Kingdom made up 6.3 per cent of the total national population (see Table 1.1). In the inner London area the overseas born were 28 per cent of the population. Nevertheless, in the 19th and 20th century many people born outside the United Kingdom have arrived and settled. The largest single immigrant and minority group throughout this period has been, and remains, the Irish. In 1861 there were 'over 600 000 Irish-born persons in England and Wales' (Krausz, 1972, p. 37). The Census for 1981 also records just over six hundred thousand persons in Great Britain born in Ireland. In the latter part of the 19th century tens of thousands of Jewish migrants came to Britain, many of them fleeing persecution and poverty in Eastern Europe and Russia. 'From 1881 to 1914', according to Krausz (1972, p. 37), 'the Jewish population rose from 65 000 to over a quarter of a million.' About 40 000 Jewish refugees settled here in the 1930s. These two groups – the Irish and Jewish – have for some time been significant minorities in Britain.

Table 1.1 Population of Great Britain, 1981 Census, Country of Birth

	All	53 556 911	
	Outside UK	3 359 825	(6.3% of all)
Of those born outside the UK:			
	– Ireland	607 428	
	– New Commonwealth	1 325 175	
	– Old Commonwealth	152 747	
	– Foreign	1 274 475	

The other two occasions of migration to Britain have been the Second World War and, since about 1950, a series of arrivals linked to the British Empire from countries which now belong to the Commonwealth group of nations. The migrants who came immediately after the Second World War were principally refugees and 'displaced persons' of whom the largest group coming to Britain were the Polish. In the late 1940s approximately 150 000 Polish people settled in Britain. Others coming in smaller numbers were Ukrainians, Baltic peoples, and Hungarians; by the 1960s there were also people settling here from Western Europe of whom the Italians (then estimated 96 000 – see Krausz, 1972, p. 35) were the largest group.

The shortage of labour in Britain in the post-war period had been one of the reasons why many European refugees were encouraged to settle here. The same is true of the slightly later migration of people from the Caribbean and from South Asia, almost all of whom were from countries which were or had been part of the British Empire – India (and Pakistan), Sri Lanka, Jamaica, Barbados, Trinidad and Guyana. People from these countries were in many cases directly recruited into labour-shortage areas of the British economy such as hospital and transport services, cotton and wool manufacture in Lancashire and Yorkshire, and heavy metal industries in the Midlands. Taken together as an overseas-born population they numbered, in 1981, 1.3 million. Those born in India (almost 400 000) were the most numerous in this 'Commonwealth' grouping, but still only two-thirds the size of the population born in Ireland which remains the largest single minority group born outside the United Kingdom. The labour force surveys for 1981–88 show the changes in total population with an overall increase of 23 per cent for all ethnic minority groups (see Table 1.2).

Racial group, ethnic group, concepts and measures

Racial group

Historically the term 'race' has had the connotations of physical type and the inheritance of characteristics both physical (typically the colour of skin) and psychosocial. The term is now discredited along with the idea that there were highly discrete divisions of humankind with determinate, inherited and unequal moral and intellectual qualities. The word race survived in the phrase 'race relations' which might better be replaced by 'ethnic relations', and in the word 'racism' which refers to the doctrine or ideology which continues to hold to the discredited ideas.

The most obvious physical difference between groups of people is the colour of skin which is indeed an inherited characteristic. Because of the social significance which is attributed to skin colour, the idea of race persists, referring to broad groups of people defined by physical appearance characteristics. 'Racial groups' are therefore not subdivisions of humankind (races) but rather groups identified by a physical characteristic, the identification being socially defined and significant and important in any number of ways. The key thing is the *social definition* not the physical characteristic.

Ethnic group

The term 'ethnic' differs from the term 'racial' because it does not have the same association with discredited theories and political ideologies. On its own it simply means 'of or associated with a people or nation'. In sociological practice it has come principally to mean a subgroup *within* a national society, where the subgroup is identified by one or more cultural signs or attributes. The principal attributes defining ethnic groups are language, religion, and real or fictive shared ancestry or

Table 1.2 Population by ethnic group, 1981–8, Great Britain

Ethnic group	Per-centage 1981	Estimated population (thousands)					Sample numbers	Percentages*	Change in population 1981–1986/88	
		1981	1986	1987	1988	1986–8 (average)	1986–8 (average)	1986–8 (average)	Thou-sands	%
West Indian†	25	528	526	489	468	495	1 340	19	0.9	− 33	− 6
African	4	80	98	116	122	112	298	4	0.2	+ 32	+ 39
Indian	35	727	784	761	814	787	2 138	31	1.4	+ 59	+ 8
Pakistani	14	284	413	392	479	428	1 169	17	0.8	+144	+ 51
Bangladeshi	2	52	117	116	91	108	289	4	0.2	+ 56	+109
Chinese	4	92	113	126	136	125	343	5	0.2	+ 33	+ 36
Arab	3	53	73	79	66	73	188	3	0.1	+ 20	+ 38
Mixed	10	217	269	263	328	287	801	11	0.5	+ 70	+ 32
Other	3	60	164	141	184	163	429	6	0.3	+103	+173
All ethnic minority groups	100	2,092	2,559	2,484	2,687	2,577	6 994	100	4.7	+485	+ 23
White	—	51,000	51,204	51,573	51,632	51,470	144 745	—	94.4	+470	+ 1
Not stated	—	608	607	467	343	472	1 540	—	0.9	−136	− 22
All ethnic groups	—	53,700	54,370	54,524	54,662	54,519	153 279	—	100.0	+819	+ 2

* Derived from grossed up estimates (column 6)
† Includes Guyanese
Averages have been calculated using unrounded figures

Sources: 1981, 1986, 1987, and 1988 Labour Force Surveys
From Haskey, 1990

historical identity (e.g. Polish Americans). The physical characteristics (e.g. colour visibility) associated with the term 'racial' and the cultural characteristics associated with the term 'ethnic' are frequently found together and overlapping. People may themselves accentuate any one characteristic as a source of identification (Black pride, Welsh speakers, followers of Islam); equally others may seize on any such characteristic in a hostile way or as a form of insult.

Table 1.3 Some definitions of ethnic groups

Note: These definitions are based on those given in Glendenning and Pearson, 1988.

Afro-Caribbean
This is a term which refers to people of African descent who were born in, or to the descendants of those who were born in, one of the islands of the Caribbean. It is preferred to 'West Indian' as this term is associated with the British imperial past

Asian
A word used to refer to persons who were born in, or whose forebears originated in, the Indian sub-continent. It refers to a wide range of persons, who between them speak several hundred languages. They do not share a single, homogeneous culture, just as 'Europeans' do not, and Afro-Caribbeans do not.

New Commonwealth
A technical term used by the Department of Health and the Department of Social Security, the Office of Population Censuses and Surveys and other government organisations. It includes the so-called 'new' Commonwealth countries (but not the 'old' (white) Commonwealth: Australia, Canada and New Zealand). Pakistan left the Commonwealth in 1972 and is included up to this date. After 1972, it is included, but as a separate entity, i.e. New Commonwealth and Pakistan (NCWP). It is often regarded as a phrase substituting for 'black'

Measures

Whilst this definition of terms is reasonably clear, the practical business of finding ways of 'measuring' group membership is by no means easy. The crude simplicities of many measures do not do justice to the complexities of the concept. But we cannot simply give up once we have decided that various kinds of information – for example, ethnic monitoring as part of an equal opportunities policy – may be valuable.

In British Census materials there are really two terms of enumeration which bear on our interest: one the enumeration of the population *by country of birth*, and two, the enumeration of the population *by the birthplace of the head of household*. Country of birth tells us too little since people born in Britain of migrant or minority group parents will themselves have many of the characteristics of so-called ethnic minority groups. To use 'birthplace of head of household' as a proxy for ethnic group membership (as is so frequently the case in many public references) rests on the unreliable assumption that where a head of household is say 'born in Jamaica' the others in that household are likely to be ethnically Jamaican or 'Afro-Caribbean'. However the figures based on this data in the 1981 Census are probably quite reasonable estimates of 'ethnic group' membership in the absence of other data (see Table 1.4). The 1991 Census will contain data based on self-assessed ethnic origin group. This question has been included after consultation with ethnic minority groups and is designed to achieve a more accurate picture of the population so that public services can be targetted more effectively where needed.

Table 1.4 Population by ethnic group (*Social Trends*, 1988, p. 26)

Total (in private households): thousands		% UK born	% of all ethnic minorities
White	51 107	96	
All ethnic minorities	2 432	43	100
West Indians	534	53	22
Indian	760	36	31
Pakistan	397	42	16
Bangladesh	103	31	4
Chinese	115	24	5
African	103	35	4
Arab	66	11	3
Mixed	235	74	10
Other	119	28	5

Source: Labour Force Survey, combined data for 1984–86

The closest we come (in official figures) to the notion of 'racial group' definitions is where 'colour' becomes the primary basis of categorisation. The term 'New Commonwealth' was really another way of defining the 'black or brown Commonwealth' since the main countries or regions making up the category are Africa, the Caribbean, and South Asia comprising India, Bangladesh, Sri Lanka and Pakistan; the familiar group of initials *NCWP* standing for New Commonwealth and Pakistan. By contrast the 'Old Commonwealth' – Australia, Canada and New Zealand – is almost like saying the 'white' Commonwealth. Particularly in the 1950s and the 1960s, rather less so now, the term 'coloured immigrants' was frequently heard and seen.

The concern with 'colour' is also evident in the annual Labour Force Surveys which 'since 1979 have included a direct question on ethnic origin' and are now 'the main source of data on ethnic minority groups in Great Britain' (Shaw, 1988). The Labour Force Survey question virtually rules out the possibility of recording 'Irish', 'Polish' or 'Jewish' (main groups mentioned above) as your ethnic origin since there is a single category – 'white':

> The Labour Force Survey question asks 'To which of the groups listed (on the card) do you consider you belong?' The categories listed are: White, West Indian, or Guyanese, Indian, Pakistani, Bangladeshi, Chinese, African, Arab, Mixed origin and other. Thus it is a self-identification question. Respondents classifying themselves as being of 'mixed' or 'other' origins are asked to describe their ethnic group in more detail and, if they then describe themselves solely in terms of one of the main categories, their replies are reclassified as appropriate. (Shaw, 1988)

The variety (of countries) allowed in what is in effect a non-white group caters in a way for the notion of ethnic origin or group membership; the single category 'white' does not allow for any differentiation in this group. We will present data from all these sources so it is important to remember how they are constructed.

Country of birth

We have noted that, in the 1981 Census, 6.3 per cent of the population were enumerated as born outside the United Kingdom. The geographical concentrations of migrants are noted by our observation that the figure for inner London is 28 per cent.

In the New Commonwealth group of countries, India and the Caribbean countries make up the largest part, but we should also note overseas born from the Far East (Hong Kong, Singapore and Malaysia) making 136 794 and Mediterranean countries (Cyprus, Gibraltar and Malta) making about 129 620 – substantial overseas-born minorities. About one half of the 1.2 million 'foreign' (i.e. not Irish or Commonwealth) born are from Europe, predominantly (373 915) European Community countries. Pakistan is the other large contributor in the 'foreign' category (188 198), although it is often presented with New Commonwealth countries, and has recently rejoined the Commonwealth.

We have seen above that the labour force survey contains an ethnic origin question distinguishing 'white' and a series of (in effect) non-white ethnic origins. These groups vary a great deal in the pattern of arrival and therefore in the proportion of that ethnic origin group who are born outside and inside the United Kingdom.

The percentage of an ethnic group which is born in the United Kingdom varies from 74 per cent (Mixed origin) to 11 per cent (Arab origin). The West Indian (apart from 'mixed') is the only group (on these definitions) which has a majority born in Britain, but other groups such as the Indian, Pakistani and Bangladeshi will approach this within the next few years as a result of births and deaths and the reduced numbers of new arrivals.

Table 1.4 shows the Indian group to be the largest single group of ethnic minorities on this definition – almost one third of the total. The South Asian group (Indian, Pakistani and Bangladeshi) make up 51 per cent of the total by contrast with the West Indian 22 per cent.

The results obtained in the 1981 Census through enumeration by birthplace of head of household correspond reasonably closely to the Labour Force Survey (1984–6) above but gives us some information that the Labour Force Survey lacks. In England and Wales the Irish population (using the head of household measure as a proxy for ethnic origin) was over 900 000. The figure for 'New Commonwealth and Pakistan' was just over 2.1 million, but also contains the important category 'East Africa'. This means persons enumerated as living in a household headed by an individual born in East Africa. Most of these would be of Indian origin and would probably classify themselves in that way in the Labour Force Survey, thus being indistinguishable from subcontinental Asians. This group was just less than 180 000 and most would be East African (Kenyan, Ugandan, Tanzanian) Asians who left or were forced out of Africa in the early 1970s. Many would be classed as refugees rather than voluntary migrants; a higher proportion of them, compared to those coming directly from India, had professional and business experience.

Some features of ethnic minority groups in the United Kingdom

Age structure

The more recently arrived ethnic minority groups (including those from the Caribbean and South Asia) have a much younger age structure than the population as a whole. The Labour Force Survey (1981–8) shows that children under 15 years of age accounted for 32 per cent of the ethnic minority population, but for only 18 per cent of the white population (see Table 1.5). Once again the undifferentiated category does not allow us to look at white ethnic minorities but the Census 'birthplace of head of household' gives some indication. The Irish group who have on average been here longer (than, say Asian and Caribbean groups) but still have considerable numbers of young new arrivals, have an age structure intermediate to (not white) ethnic minorities and 'whites', one in four being under the age of 16. Other minority groups (such as Polish and Italian) for whom there is no age data, will have much older age structures than the Caribbean and Asian groups.

The opposite side of the picture is that some ethnic minorities will have amongst them very few older people. Some but not all – because, for example, those adult Polish refugees who came to the United Kingdom in the 1940s are now quite an old population. Those who came as young adults from the Caribbean from 1949 onwards (a large proportion coming between 1957 and 1961) are now in their sixties and seventies and quite numerous. In the New Commonwealth population only about 4 per cent (in 1981) were over pensionable age, compared with approximately 20 per cent in the population as a whole. But this proportion will grow quite quickly and within a decade or so the age structure of most of these minority groups will be close to that of the whole population.

We can see in Table 1.5, containing data from the Labour Force Surveys (1981–8) that the earlier-arriving West Indian origin population includes 7 per cent who are 60 years or older, compared with only 2 per cent in the recently arrived Bangladeshi population. Furthermore, in the next age group down (45–59 years) the West Indian population is similar to the white (20 per cent and 17 per cent). Many of this section of the minority group population – West Indians in their fifties – will soon be in their sixties and swelling the size of the elderly Afro-Caribbean population. This has many implications for social policies and services for the elderly, many of which are discussed in Fenton (1987), *Ageing Minorities*. Most of the elderly Caribbean people in Britain are those who have grown old here over the last 40 years. This ageing is also occurring in the (on average) slightly later arriving Asian population, but in this group there are also elderly people who have come as dependants of sons and daughters settled here. The important point is that in these groups there are elderly people who have been here a long time, and elderly people who have been here a very short time. Their physical, social, cultural and psychological needs may be quite different in nature – or at least in emphasis.

Geographical distribution

Groups migrating to a new country are almost always unevenly distributed geographically. The Irish in Britain are largely an urban population, particularly in London and western port cities such as Liverpool and Bristol, but many came in search of agricultural work originally, before the urbanisation of so much farmland. Jewish people arriving in Britain also settled in port towns (including of course London) but many of them moved on into such large industrial and commercial centres as Leeds and Manchester.

People arriving from the Caribbean in the 1950s also settled in some areas much more than others: London attracted many immigrants and today a high proportion of all Britain's Caribbean ethnic minority group live in London and the South East. Other areas of settlement include the Midlands (e.g. Birmingham, Wolverhampton), Manchester, Leeds and Bristol.

Table 1.5 Population by age and ethnic group, 1986–8, Great Britain

percentages

Ethnic group	Age-group											All ages		Males per 100 females
	Under 1	1–4	5–9	10–14	15–19	20–24	25–34	35–44	45–59	60 and over age*	Pen-sionable	%	Thou-sands	
West Indian†	2	8	7	7	10	14	16	9	20	7	5	100	495	94
African	(2)	8	8	8	8	13	20	17	12	3	(2)	100	112	120
Indian	2	9	10	8	9	10	20	14	14	5	4	100	787	100
Pakistani	2	13	15	11	10	9	16	10	11	2	2	100	428	107
Bangladeshi	3	17	14	13	9	7	15	8	13	2	(1)	100	108	124
Chinese	(1)	7	10	10	8	9	23	18	9	5	4	100	125	101
Arab	(2)	8	7	(4)	5	12	28	17	11	6	(4)	100	73	163
Mixed	5	18	17	12	13	10	11	7	6	3	3	100	287	93
Other	2	9	9	7	7	10	20	18	11	6	5	100	163	100
All ethnic minority groups	2	10	11	9	10	10	18	12	13	5	4	100	2 577	102
White	1	5	6	6	7	8	14	14	17	21	19	100	51 470	95
Not stated	3	7	8	9	9	9	14	12	13	18	16	100	472	95
All ethnic groups	1	5	6	6	8	8	14	14	16	20	18	100	54 519	95

* 65 and over for men, 60 and over for women
† Includes Guyanese
Figures in brackets are based on a sample of fewer than 30

Sources: 1986, 1987 and 1988 Labour Force Surveys
From Haskey, 1990

Table 1.6 New Commonwealth ethnic minority groups in Greater London and in England and Wales. 1981 Census. Population by birthplace of head of household

Ethnic Group (birthplace of Head of Household)	England and Wales	Greater London
UK born	43 598 565	4 837 904
Irish	907 013	300 621
Caribbean	544 236	306 792
Indian	657 563	223 664
All NCWP	2 161 057	945 148

Source: Census reports for Great Britain and Greater London (Table 11)

Table 1.6 shows that one in ten UK-born people live in Greater London, compared with one in three Irish, almost three in five Caribbean, and one in three Indian people (by the birthplace of head of household measure). South Asian migrants have also settled in London and the South East. Beyond this area considerable settlement of Asians can be found in the East Midlands (particularly Leicester) and in the Lancashire and Yorkshire cotton and wool towns. These are also settlements of *particular* groups – of Sikhs in Southall, Muslims in Bradford and Gujeratis in Leicester. Furthermore within these towns and cities there will usually be particular areas of concentration. For example about one half of Bristol's ethnic minority population lives in four of the city's thirty-plus wards. Within these wards (which may have up to 30 per cent ethnic minority population against 4 per cent for Bristol as a whole) there will be smaller areas where the ethnic minority population may be 50 per cent or more of that small area (often an 'enumeration district' is the base of recording). In such cases it should perhaps be asked, 'who is the real ethnic minority?' These patterns of geographical distribution have obvious implications for the provision and planning of services.

Health, housing, education and employment

In a short chapter such as this it is impossible to say much about these major institutional areas. Readers should look at source books such as *Britain's Black Population* (1988, Radical Statistics Race Group – Bhat et al.) and *Black and White Britain* (Brown, 1984) and refer to the Commission for Racial Equality pamphlets and booklets, especially where they focus on a special issue such as discrimination in the allocation of council housing.

As in all areas the overrepresentation of ethnic minorities in poorer socioeconomic classes means that they share with other poorer people the experience of inadequate housing, low incomes and unhealthy environmental conditions. But then ethnic minorities are not exclusively concentrated in lower socioeconomic classes. Racial discrimination, and class and racial disadvantage cannot be ignored in understanding the position of ethnic minorities. At the same time it should not be thought that 'ethnic minorities' are 'mere victims' of external circumstances. In housing, education and employment the pattern is in many respects similar. Black people in Britain have had the experiences typical of their social class position and 'partake' of many of the familiar inequalities. At the same time they have experienced the particular results of racial hostility, racist attitudes and discriminatory practices. In housing, for example, working class Afro-Caribbean people have struggled to find decent housing just as white working class families may do. But *within* a largely working class market for council housing Afro-Caribbean people have been allocated much of the worst housing available, either through direct or indirect discriminatory practices. In education most studies appear to show that young black people – specifically *males* – do not achieve as good results at school as their white or Asian counterparts. But there is a great deal of dispute as to why, and to what extent, this is the case. Caribbean and Asian British young people are just now beginning to appear in considerable numbers in higher education but it is probable that they are still under-represented. Several studies have demonstrated both disadvantage and discrimination in the access of ethnic minority youngsters to Youth Training Schemes.

In employment, the patterns of migration to which we have alluded developed out of the movement of successive groups of migrants into particular *niches* in the economy. Often they have entered occupations which (in a period of labour shortage) indigenous workers had abandoned, and have worked under less desirable conditions (for example, in the most physically demanding jobs, in shifts, in insecure forms of employment). As South Asian women have increasingly entered the job market they are vulnerable to various forms of super-exploitation some of which have been documented. At the same time, as we mentioned above, some ethnic minority individuals and families have achieved considerable, if not great, wealth by their professional and business expertise. The 1984 Policy Studies Institute Review (Brown, 1984) concluded that 'overall the job levels of whites are much higher than those of Asians and West Indians, but there is considerable variation between men and women, and between the different sections of the black population' (p. 157).

This picture of over-representation of ethnic minority groups in lower socioeconomic groups has been broadly true through recent decades but some of the most recent data suggests that either this is less true now than used to be the case or the difference between sub-groups *within* the ethnic minorities and the differences between men and women are more significant than has been recognised.

In Table 1.7 we can see that, looking at (in the survey's own terms) 'white' and 'non-white' groups overall, the differences favour the white group but not by a very large amount. Among men, 26 per cent of whites are in professional and managerial employment, compared with 23 per cent of non-white men. Seventeen per cent of white men are in semi-skilled or unskilled occupations, compared with 25 per cent of non-whites. But the differences *within* these categories are much more striking. While 26 per cent of white men are in the first two socioeconomic groups, the percentage of Indian ethnic origin men is 29 per cent, and for West Indian origin men 7 per cent. Furthermore, while 54 per cent of white men are in the three (skilled, semi-skilled and unskilled) manual categories, the percentage for West Indian men is 74 per cent and for Indians 54 per cent. But among women, 29 per cent of those of Indian origin are in semi-skilled occupations compared with only 21 per cent of all women. One reason why this relationship of those of Indian origin to all others has been obscured is the practice of presenting all 'Asians' together. The more recently arrived Pakistanis and Bangladeshis are over-represented in the skilled, semi-skilled and unskilled manual categories.

Table 1.7 Socioeconomic group by ethnic origin and sex, Great Britain, 1987

Socioeconomic group and sex	Ethnic group							Percentages
	White	All ethnic minority groups	West Indian or Guyanese	Indian	Pakistani or Bangladeshi	Other (incl. Mixed ethnic groups)	Not stated	All groups
Men								
Professional	7	9	2	14	5	11	9	7
Employers, managers	19	14	5	15	14	20	19	19
Other non-manual	18	17	17	16	10	21	18	18
Skilled manual	37	34	43	35	35	25	36	37
Semi-skilled manual	13	20	21	16	31	17	14	14
Unskilled manual	4	5	10	3	5	4	3	4
Armed forces/inadequately described/not stated	1	1	1	0	—	3	1	1
All groups (thousands=100%)	**13 201**	**501**	**113**	**171**	**82**	**135**	**124**	**13 825**
Women								
Professional	1	2	1	4	—	3	2	1
Employers, managers	9	6	3	6	—	8	8	8
Other non-manual	53	50	55	44	—	51	57	53
Skilled manual	8	10	5	15	—	8	8	8
Semi-skilled manual	21	26	27	29	—	22	18	21
Unskilled manual	7	6	8	3	—	7	7	7
Armed forces/inadequately described/not stated	—	—	—	—	—	1	—	0
All groups (thousands=100%)	**9 614**	**327**	**114**	**109**	**15**	**89**	**103**	**10 044**

Source: Labour Force Survey 1987 (1989).

Immigration, discrimination and Europe

The arrival of New Commonwealth-origin migrants to this country has been governed by a series of immigration laws and regulations. Racially hostile and indeed *racist* attitudes have been expressed and confirmed by these laws which have progressively closed the door on non-white immigration to Britain. A 'firm' immigration policy is seen by many as one which keeps 'black people out'. This partly reflects racist attitudes in the public; in part governments and politicians, from Powell to Tebbit, have encouraged and confirmed these attitudes by their statements and postures. The fact that such familiar statements are made in the 1990s about migration from Hong Kong reminds us that nothing has changed much in this respect. In the 1970s the National Front threatened to promote such attitudes electorally (as well as on the streets); their weakness since can largely be attributed to the Conservatives' wooing back their supporters by appealing to similar sentiments.

The increasingly harsh and restrictive immigration laws and procedures have done untold damage to the lives of black people in Britain. Women have been arbitrarily and unnecessarily subjected to vaginal examinations at airports – their introduction to British society. Thousands of *bona fide* visitors – particularly from Jamaica – are turned away when they have come to attend weddings or funerals in this country. The rate of rejection of black visitors is much higher than for other groups of visitors. Many commentators fear that the expected new frontier arrangements after 1992 within the European Community will adversely affect all minorities within Europe, including black British citizens. The best single source on this topic is Gordon (1969), *Fortress Europe? The Meaning of 1992* which expresses fears about a rising tide of racism in Europe. The changes anticipated in 1992, concludes Gordon, are likely to diminish yet further Britain's commitment to people from the Commonwealth and threaten the citizenship rights of Britain's black ethnic minority groups. In addition, there may be an increase in migration, especially of unskilled workers, to the inner cities (NETRHA, 1990).

The main legal instrument designed to use the law against racial discrimination is the 1976 Race Relations Act which created the Commission for Racial Equality (CRE) to carry out the intentions of the Act. As a very brief summary, the broadly agreed conclusions are:

1. despite some weaknesses, the Act provides the legal instruments to combat discrimination;
2. the Commission has been greatly weakened by lack of resources and political support;
3. 'Racial discrimination 17 years after the Act' (a study by the Policy Studies Institute) shows that there has been no measurable diminution in acts of racial discrimination, indeed they may have increased.

The authors concluded that two major reasons for this were, firstly, that employers who discriminated had little reason to fear being found out or face legal action and, secondly, the under-resourcing of the CRE. Living in cultural groups may be a response to racial attack, but admission to institutions denies that response.

Positive change

In many ways those who wish to combat discrimination, disadvantage and racism know *what* needs to be done; the need is for *resources* and *political will*. In the provision of health and social services, at the local level, many people have given time and effort to reconsidering their work in the context of a multi-ethnic society. The work done at this level should be valued and continued, even though all these services face the widespread cuts in funding that have so damaged the whole health and welfare sector in the last decade. The provision of advocacy and linkworker schemes in health centres have been very valuable; the slow but important recognition that mental health services need to be reformed, if they are to meet fully the needs of minority group patients, shows another way forward in a positive direction.

We should also be made aware of how voluntary groups have inspired the development of services which were unlikely ever to have come from the statutory sector. These are often, by their very nature, responsive to local needs and sentiments, and an example is described in Chapter 6. The great weakness of this sector, however, is the uncertainty of funding; if many of these groups could be placed on a more secure financial footing without losing their local responsiveness much would be gained.

Local authorities have played an important part in developing equal opportunities policies with reference both to employment and to the provision of services. In some cases this has led to real gains in the quality of services available to ethnic minority people. However in the same period there has been a significant attack by central government on local democracy which has weakened local authorities politically and financially. Indeed the most significant change which could be made to improve the quality of life of ethnic minorities in Britain would be an expression of political will from the centre which could signify the commitment of the whole society to racial justice.

References

BHAT, A., CARR-HILL, R. and OHRI, S. (1988). *Britain's Black Population*, 2nd edn. Gower (for The Radical Statistics Race Group), Aldershot.

BROWN, C. (Policy Studies Institute) (1984). *Black and White Britain*. Heinemann, London.

BROWN, C. and GAY, P. (1985). *Racial Discrimination 17 Years after the Act*. Policy Studies Institute, London.

FENTON, S. (1987). *Ageing Minorities*. Commission for Racial Equality, London.

GLENDENNING, F. and PEARSON, M. (1988). *Black and Ethnic Minority Elders in Britain: Health Needs and Access to Services*. Health Education Authority, London/Centre for Social Gerontology, University of Keele.

GORDON, P. (1969). *Fortress Europe. The Meaning of 1992*. The Runnymede Trust, Princelet Street, London.

HASKEY, J. (1990). The ethnic minority populations of Great Britain: estimates by ethnic group and country of birth. *Population Trends*, No. 60: pp. 35–8.

KRAUSZ, E. (1972). *Ethnic Minorities in Britain*. Paladin, London.

NETRHA (1990). *Health Services for People from Ethnic Minorities. A Report on a conference organised by North East Thames Regional Health Authority.* NETRHA, London.

RADICAL STATISTICS RACE GROUP (1988). *Britain's Black Population*, 2nd edn. Gower, Aldershot.

SHAW, C. (1988). Estimates of ethnic minority populations, *Population Trends*, No. 51: pp. 5–8.

2

History of migration to the United Kingdom

John Young and James George

The latter half of the 20th century has brought a very real sense of global shrinking. Major components have been ease of travel, improved communication systems and the electronic news media. But migration of people, as individuals or as groups, has had a powerful additional effect on exchanging cultures and broadening horizons. Seeking out a 'cause' or a 'reason' for a particular migration is problematic. One helpful approach which, at least to some extent, can be applied as an explanatory model is the notion of 'pull/push' factors.

Pushed situation

The pushed group would be characteristic of the refugee. Some refugees are political and others economic, but both groups effectively seek to escape from intolerable personal circumstances within their own country. Such groups have entered Britain in a state of desperation, with few possessions, financial resources or clear plan for the future. Some may be in family units; others may have left important family members behind with no realistic hope of establishing regular contact with them again. They all carry with them mixed, perhaps confused, memories and are often poorly equipped emotionally to adjust and thrive in a new culture. We need only to reflect on how we personally would be affected if forced away from our home, neighbourhood, friends, family and work into a land where the language and customs were new and where we were regarded as foreigners. It is not surprising, therefore, that psychological scars may develop centred around people, places and lifestyles left behind, which cannot be recaptured other than in reflective, introspective moments. Such refugees may fall into a time trap, recalling life as it *was* but knowing that time has marched on with fundamental changes occurring in their homeland from which they now feel estranged. They may be unable, therefore, to integrate fully while no longer feeling that they belong to their country of origin.

Case history 1: Mrs Kajando

Mrs Kajando is an Estonian lady living in the United Kingdom. She is now nearly 90 years old having fled Estonia when it was annexed into the Soviet Union. In Estonia, she was a woman of substance and education. Fear of Stalin's purges forced her and her husband first to Germany then, via France, to Britain. She speaks Estonian, Russian, Polish, German, French and English. Her husband died 15 years ago and her small group of Estonian emigrés have slowly dwindled. She remains a lady full of poise and pride but has no sense of purpose or belonging. She feels Estonian but recognises that her homeland, as she knew it, is no more. (It has been heavily dominated by Russian culture; 40 per cent of the inhabitants are now Russian.) A small part of her is demanding to return, but for the most part she has no wish to do so: she has an intense fear of revisiting a country now perceived as a foreign land, and undergoing yet further change. These turmoils and cultural loneliness have led to despondency and frank depression at times. Her children have been born and raised in the United Kingdom and, although sympathetic and supportive, they are unable to share her past or understand her perplexity. Her old age has become a suffering.

Pulled situation

The opposite component of the push-pull model, the pull factors, operates where an individual or group have been attracted to Britain for self-betterment and (usually) a potentially more prosperous way of life. The best contemporary example here is the migration of the South Asians from the Indian sub-continent. In the main these represent people who had a reasonably satisfactory way of life but saw greater prospects for training and earnings in Britain. It has been common for one member of the family, usually the son, to migrate sometimes followed at a later stage by his wife, children and parents. This has led to difficulties for many of these people as they have retained a strong home orientation with a feeling of being outposted for a flexible but limited period in a foreign country. They maintain a fall back position of the sanctuary of their own homeland and close contact with their families to whom many send financial assistance at regular intervals. Most adapt well to being split between two continents. For some, however, tensions develop through a resettlement trap in which the second generation sons and their wives stand between the two cultures. The third generation children become closely integrated into the local culture and British way of life, but the first generation parents have greatest difficulties in integrating and generally remain separate in compact Asian communities. Such competing loyalties and orientations may produce latent conflicts which are stored up to be released at times of ill health.

Case history 2: Mr Singh

Mr Nassim Singh, an 86-year-old Sikh gentleman, was admitted to hospital following a hemiplegic stroke. He had suffered an earlier stroke six months previously from which he had made an almost complete recovery. He had retained a now prosperous farm in the Punjab with a big house and staff where his younger son still lived with his own family. He had sent his older son to Britain some 20 years previously for 'commercial reasons'. He had followed after eight years but had made frequent return journeys to his farm. The second stroke had left him disabled to the extent that he needed more care and attention than could be provided by his working son and daughter-in-law. Their own children had been wholly brought up and educated in Britain. In the light of his new disabilities, he decided that he and his complete extended family should return to the Punjab. This suggestion provoked great distress on the part of his son in Britain who, whilst recognising the authority of his father, faced strong objections from his own children who rebelled and refused to contemplate a new life in the Punjab. He was caught between a loyalty to his father and a commitment to his children's happiness.

Elderly people of Afro-Caribbean origin

The great majority of elderly people from the West Indies came to the United Kingdom in the boom period after the Second World War. However, Britain and the Caribbean Islands have had a close association for nearly three centuries. Initially, this was through trade with the financially successful 17th century triangular trading route between Britain, the African Coast, and the Caribbean Islands, with the infamous middle passage of slave carriage to the islands. Later, the sugar plantations of Jamaica, Barbados, Trinidad and other islands of the British West Indies were under direct rule as part of the British Empire. The islanders were therefore imbued with British values and surrounded by Empire trappings. There was a strong feeling of identity with the 'mother country' which was reinforced by an educational system which strongly emphasised a sanitised version of British society. For the better educated and ambitious, however, there were few opportunities for advancement as middle and top civil service posts were occupied by graduate career diplomats from Britain. A restlessness developed based in part on self-betterment, and in part on a desire to visit the 'mother country'.

The Second World War provided an important opportunity for many to realise their ambitions. The hunger for labour to drive the war machine in Britain stimulated a Caribbean labour recruitment campaign. Several thousand joined the RAF and were trained as engineers and mechanics. These people found themselves reluctantly repatriated after demobilisation: many would have preferred to stay. They returned to a deteriorating Caribbean economy which was dependent on sugar exports and suffered greatly during a commodity price collapse. There was escalating unemployment and general despair. Prospects of self betterment in Britain seemed obvious. There was also a sense of adventure – almost a pilgrimage to the centre of the Empire which was fuelled by encouraging stories from the repatriated ex-servicemen.

The start of the post-war Caribbean population migration is usually attributed to the docking at Tilbury on 22 June 1948 of an old troop carrier called the 'Empire Windrush' (Fig. 2.1). It was much publicised at the time. Some 500 Jamaicans suffered the uncomfortable journey; many were returning ex-RAF servicemen but there was a rude shock for others with their first sighting of dirty streets, slums and ruins and early experience of the British uncharitable weather.

In the ten years following the arrival of the 'Empire Windrush', 125 000 West Indians came to Britain. Up to a quarter were highly trained with professional and managerial skills. These people had the greatest difficulty in obtaining work in a Britain that was poorly prepared to receive an influx of black workers. Their arrival rapidly exposed latent racism within British society. There was much political confusion engendered on the one hand by a fear of 'open access' for all Commonwealth citizens, and on the other the need for extra labour to satisfy a rampant expanding economy with production increases of 8 per cent per annum at

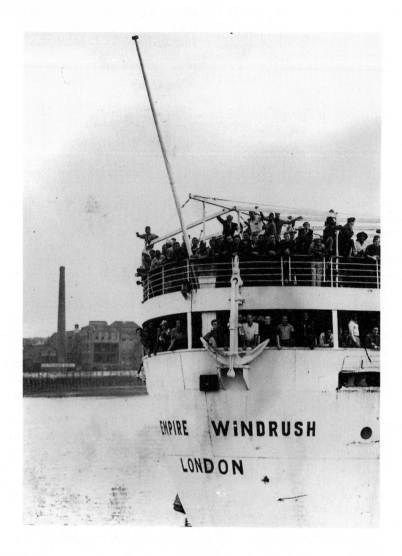

Fig. 2.1 The 'Empire Windrush' bringing 482 Jamaicans to Britain.

this time. In the event, so acute was the labour shortage that policy was dictated by the pressing practical needs of the day and active immigration from the West Indies was encouraged by a recruitment drive and assisted passage (Fig. 2.2). Most of the new arrivals worked in public transport or the health service, with a smaller number in manufacturing. Many intended originally to return home with proof of their success. Return without it would be a sign of failure which some could not consider.

As with the Irish and the South Asians, migration was predominantly from villages and a new conurbation life required considerable adjustment. It is important

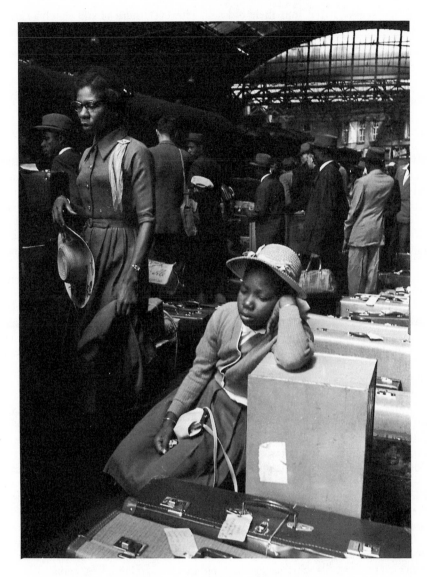

Fig. 2.2 Newly arrived immigrants at Victoria Station.

to remember, too, that there are very distinct differences in culture and previous eperience between people from different islands in the Caribbean. Over half the West Indians who came to Britain came from Jamaica: others came from Guyana, Barbados, Trinidad and Tobago. Those from the island of Dominica had a colonial heritage which was French. Many West Indians are Christians; the largest group are Pentecostalists, some are Anglicans or Baptists and a few are Methodists or Roman Catholics. It has been from this background that the ethnic Caribbean elders have emerged. For many there have been strong feelings of disappointment and sadness, with life scars carried into their old age. However there is still much pride in their background and an independence of spirit which sustains them in times of ill health.

East African Asians

These settlers came to Britain from Uganda, Kenya, and Tanzania in the late 1970s and early 1980s. They constitute a distinctive group of Asian settlers in that they are 'twice removed' having originally left India during the early part of the 20th century as indentured labour to build the Kenya/Uganda railways. This first intercontinental journey had been stimulated by the prospect of financial self-improvement. Many of these Asians remained in the East African countries forming the administrative and operative personnel of the railways they had helped build. They had predominantly occupied East African townships where they formed isolated pocket communities. But it was this isolation which led to their displacement following independence for the East African colonies. The Asian labour force had provided highly skilled personnel, both middle level administrators and professionals. Independence of the African countries was followed by a policy of Africanisation which most affected the public services and was felt especially strongly by the South Asians. As the process of Africanisation accelerated, Asians working in the civil service were sacked and the political climate was such that private firms were reluctant to take them on. These circumstances led to the migration of South Asians to countries abroad. For the Ugandan Asians, the displacement was far more acute when, in short order, they were ousted by the policies of General Amin in 1972.

Although the East African Asians are distinguished by their common background of 'twice migrated', this common background should not obscure the several different cultures contained within this apparently homogenous group. There are Hindus, Muslims, Gujeraties and Sikhs. Within this caveat, however, many East African Asians do share certain common features which distinguish and set them aside from Asians migrating to Britain directly from the Indian subcontinent. Firstly, they had a long established urban background and were familiar with town life in contrast to the mainly rural Asians from the Indian subcontinent. They brought with them a range of managerial and professional skills. They were also relatively prosperous and had a certain amount of capital which freed them from the poor quality housing occupied by many immigrants in the United Kingdom and provided them with a more secure foothold in a foreign land. This meant that they were more able to establish themselves in successful small businesses. The effect of being 'twice migrated' produced a feeling of confidence from collective and individual experience from the first migration. There was also a freeing from the 'myth of return': the stance which migrant groups can take up when a bridge to their homeland persists which can counter feelings of alienation. For the East African Asians there was no such fall back refuge: it was Britain or nowhere. This certainly concentrated the mind and promoted a greater wish for integration and a more positive orientation towards mainstream British society. They also had the benefit of migrating as whole family units. Clearly this produced a potential for much increased personal strength and mutual support and is in sharp contrast to the

Indian sub-continent Asian experience. Here it was largely individuals who migrated, rather like expeditionaries attempting to find a foothold and, perhaps at a later stage, being joined by their families.

Elderly people of Vietnamese origin

Vietnamese refugees are recent migrants. Since the Communist victory in Vietnam, and the subsequent unification of that country in 1975, several thousand Vietnamese refugees have been resettled in Britain. The majority come from North Vietnam and most are ethnic Chinese who speak both Cantonese and Vietnamese. Most of those who arrived in Britain came from reception camps in Hong Kong which were established to provide temporary shelter for this group of so called 'boat people'. It was racial persecution which stimulated the exodus from Vietnam. The new Vietnam administration became increasingly dependent on the Soviet Union whereas China started to forge stronger ties with the United States. Relations between Vietnam and China were therefore strained and the Hanoi regime sought to present its ethnic Chinese population as insidious agents of Peking. They became persecuted with withdrawal of work permits, ration cards and closure of their schools. Life became intolerable.

For many, the exodus was desperate and harrowing in small overcrowded boats with little food and few personal possessions. They spent varying time in cramped reception centres in Hong Kong before dispersing mostly to Britain or America.

On arrival in Britain the refugees spent between three months and one year in reception centres. Here they learnt about the British way of life, were taught English and were prepared for resettlement. Unfortunately the resettlement programme was of necessity rather rushed and difficulties emerged. In the main, the Vietnamese refugees had a rural background with little formal education. Learning a new language and culture represented an ambitious task and many left the reception centres only poorly equipped to cope with their new environment and with a less than adequate grasp of the English language. A further factor was that of 'displacement shock': many refugees being psychologically ill-prepared following their fraught and dangerous exodus. There was the additional tension of coming to terms with an uncertain future in a hugely different culture, and the inbred fear of 'government' buildings – including hospitals.

Unfortunately, there was not sufficient vacant housing in any one local authority in Britain to accommodate significantly large groups of Vietnamese families. Rather, they were dispersed throughout small towns in the United Kingdom in small groups of four to ten families. They were therefore denied the mutual support of small local communities of fellow countrymen. In this respect they differ from other ethnic minority groups such as the South Asians or some of the Middle European settlers such as the Poles. Unfortunately also, they arrived on the employment scene just as unemployment reached its highest. Their employment backgrounds were rural, many being fishermen or farmers. Others were craftsmen but with skills that were not in high demand – silversmiths and jewellers for example. Not surprisingly, those who found work mainly found unskilled jobs such as hospital auxiliaries, store keepers and night watchmen.

Elderly Chinese

Large scale migration of Chinese to Britain is quite recent compared with the number of Chinese who left for the Americas, Australia and South East Asia as 'coolies' and contract labourers in the 19th century. The vast majority have come from Hong Kong and therefore differ from earlier migrants who predominantly originated from the Chinese provinces of Gwandong and Fujina. The late 19th century Chinese were forced out by the oppressive regime of the last Manchu emperors.

The earliest Chinese arrivals at the end of the last century contained a significant proportion who were fleeing American persecution as they were driven from their homes in California. Other Chinese entered Britain after jumping ship seeking better paid work. Some continued to work in the dockland areas but increasingly the Chinese became associated with the laundry trade. These Chinese immigrants were principally seeking rapid accumulation of wealth before returning home to Southern China. Setting up a laundry required little capital but involved great physical toil. They established the early Chinatowns in London, Manchester and Liverpool.

The much larger scale Chinese immigration took place in the 1950s and 1960s. It was stimulated by a great enthusiasm and fashion for Chinese food and a rapid expansion in the Chinese restaurant trade. Many of the Hong Kong Chinese who came to Britain at this time relied on contacts already established here to find employment. These contacts were often brothers, uncles, cousins, fellow villagers or friends. Family emigration took place in stages over several years. Many of the Chinese elders, therefore, may be fairly recent emigrants who came to join their sons and daughters. They may encounter considerable difficulties adapting to a new culture compounded by language and literacy problems and ill health due to a life time of work in kitchens or on the land. The Hong Kong Chinese community in Britain is widely scattered, working mainly in Chinese restaurants in almost every town in Britain. The larger communities are in London, Cardiff, Manchester, Burnley and Liverpool.

Elderly people of Cypriot origin

The first major group of Cypriots, who are mainly Greek speaking, came during the 1930s and worked predominantly in the clothing industries.

In the late 1950s and early 1960s further Greek and Turkish Cypriots came to Britain for work or to escape the political situation in Cyprus. After the crisis in 1974, Cypriot residents were joined by thousands of homeless relatives. The majority of Cypriots have settled in London. Many are now elderly and, although literate in Greek or Turkish, may be unable to cope with spoken English and have become socially isolated.

Elderly people of Central and Eastern European origin

Jewish refugees from Russia and Rumania came to Britain to escape persecution at the end of the 19th and the beginning of the 20th century. The influx was numerically very large and was particularly noticeable because of the rather small numbers of Jewish people living in Britain before this time. These new immigrants were a culturally distinct section of the Jewish people who spoke Yiddish and were concentrated in a limited range of workshop trades rather than the familiar shopkeeper and merchant role. Many had had the original intent of reaching the expanding North Americas and had intended to use Britain as a staging point but settled here instead. They settled predominantly in the East End of London, and in Leeds and Manchester. Further Jewish refugees came to settle in Britain to escape Nazi persecution.

After the Second World War, large numbers of people from Cental and Eastern Europe were actively recruited by the government to work in British industry. Apart from the Poles, these included Ukraines, Czechs, Rumanians, Germans, Yugoslavs, Estonians and Latvians. Subsequently, almost 20,000 new-comers arrived from Hungary after the 1956 unrest. Many of these people are now elderly and speak little English. Many have a deep sense of exile. The Eastern European elderly are by no means a homogenous group, having several different cultures and religions. They may be Jewish or alternatively belong to many Christian denominations including Orthodox, Roman Catholic, or Lutheran.

South Asians from the Indian subcontinent

There is a long established tradition of migration from the Indian subcontinent to a wide scatter of countries. For example, between 1834 and 1937 the total migration from India has been estimated at approximately 30 million, but, of these, 24 million returned leaving only 6 million as permanent migrants. This pattern of essentially short term migration has persisted. Much of this early migration was for indentured or contract labour and only within the British Empire, as it then was. East and South Africa, the West Indies, and South East Asia, particularly Malaya and parts of Borneo, have considerable settlements of Indians. Subsequently, political and social changes closed many of these old migration inlets. Demographic, economic and, in some cases, political developments in the Indian subcontinent continued however and increased in intensity as factors pushing towards emigration. After 1955, migrants from India and Pakistan began to enter Britain in increasing numbers They came from the Punjab, particularly districts of Jullundar and Hoshiarpur, and from the central and southern parts of Gujerat. From the West Punjab in Pakistan, the northwest frontier area and Mirpur district of Kashmir, and the Sylhet district of Bangladesh. This wide scatter of small geographical pockets of migration sources can be seen in Fig. 2.3. These migrants comprise widely different cultural, religious and language backgrounds as indicated in Table 2.1.

The factors underlying the stimulus for emigration of these various groups are very mixed. Undoubtedly, however, the established tradition of migration for people living in these areas has acted as an influential backdrop. The Sikhs of Punjab, in

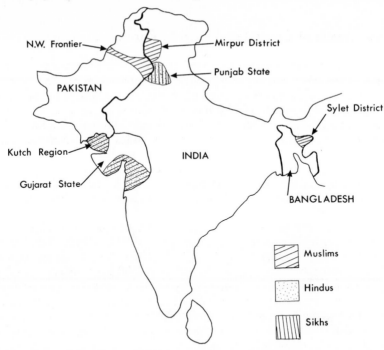

Fig. 2.3 Diagram showing the major areas of the Indian subcontinent from which people have emigrated to the United Kingdom.

Table 2.1 Asians in the United Kingdom

Country of Origin	Province of Origin	Language	Main Religion
India	Punjab	Punjabi/Hindi/Urdu	Sikhism
	Gujarat	Gujarati	Hinduism
Pakistan	Punjab	Punjabi/Hindi/Urdu	
	Mirpur	Mirpuri/Punjabi	Islam
	North West Frontier	Pashto/Punjabi/Urdu	
Bangladesh	Sylhet	Bengali (Sylheti dialect)	Islam
Africa Kenya Tanzania Uganda Malawi	Majority from Gujarat	Gujarati/Punjabi/ English/Swahili	Hinduism Sikhism and Islam

particular, have proven themselves to be the most adventurous of Indian migrants and are now widely dispersed in many parts of the world. It has been this venturesome spirit which has been the main driving force for these Sikhs drawing them away from their Punjab homeland. For the people of Bangladesh also, there is an established acceptance of travel and wandering. They are a seafaring nation and many were driven by poverty and drawn by ambition to leave their homes at an early age and to work in the merchant ships of the Raj. Some settled in the cities of Britain where their presence has been the stimulus for further migration, from the Sylhet district in particular. Many well educated people from Pakistan and Bangladesh followed a tradition of obtaining higher British qualifications to gain top level jobs at home. Most returned but some stayed behind or returned after brief visits to their homeland where they were not fully satisfied with their way of life. The break up of East Pakistan in 1971, resulting in the birth of Bangladesh, was a major factor in a much larger wave of migration. At this time 'push' factors due to political uncertainties, unstable economy, and poor job opportunities took precedence over the previous 'pull' factors. The settlers entering Britain at this time (and also large numbers to other European countries, the USA and Canada) were essentially economic refugees escaping from an uncertain rural life and farming and seeking a more prosperous standard of living in industrial work in Britain. Most of these settlers have retained strong links with their homeland and indeed many have returned upon retirement.

Elderly people of Irish origin

There was a major influx of Irish migrants, particularly in the 1920s and 1930s, many from rural areas. The men took up labouring and navvying jobs and the women tended to be employed in domestic service. Many of the men were employed 'on the lump' with wages being paid in cash and they were encouraged to avoid tax and insurance. Many of their employers took no interest in the welfare of their workforce and working conditions were hard with illness and industrial accidents common. Lack of proper employment, insurance and tax records often prevented these people from claiming welfare benefits. Many lived in poor housing conditions in inner cities on inadequate diets. These difficulties have often followed elderly Irish people into old age resulting in poor mental and physical health.

Conclusion

The post-war industrial prosperity in Britain has provided the general backdrop attracting a diverse range of migrant settlers. Several of the larger groups have been discussed above but there are many numerically smaller but equally important settlers who have not been included. Many of these people are now entering old age when ill health becomes an increasing threat. Neglect of previous background and culture, and of the circumstances stimulating the migration are particularly detrimental during illness when trust, empathy and openness may become jeopardised by unintended misunderstandings. A little extra time and patience may be all that is required to avoid this outcome.

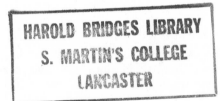

3

A place to stay: growing old away from home

Pam Schweitzer

Reminiscence: the work of Age Exchange

Reminiscence is a natural and enjoyable activity in old age enabling people to take stock of their lives. It provides an equally important function of sharing those memories with younger generations to give a sense of history of their culture. When people are away from their homelands, this natural process is hampered and arrangements for it to occur have to be created. This need was addressed in 1983 with the creation of Age Exchange as a reminiscence theatre and publishing company, and a registered charity based in South East London. Age Exchange creates professional theatre productions from the reminiscences and current concerns of older people in the London area, touring these shows widely to stimulate further reminiscence on the part of audiences. The research material collected for these shows is published in book form so that there is a lasting record of the life experience of those who contribute their recollections.

In Autumn 1990, Age Exchange Reminiscence Centre hosted the first National Conference on Multicultural Reminiscence. With a full take up of places by people from many different fields such as health, education, social services, library services and the arts, the conference demonstrated that there is a great deal of interest in the field of reminiscence with ethnic elders and an urgent need for more resources to be made available.

Collecting reminiscences

Sometimes the gleaning of these stories is a group activity, where several elderly people meet together with a reminiscence worker who will stimulate their memories with photographs and artifacts and carefully prepared questions. As the elderly people listen to each other, they remember more of their own experiences, some of which may have been forgotten for many years. The experience of working in this way with a group of other people who have related experience is highly enjoyable and very reassuring. People feel more confident and less isolated when they are finding common ground and relaying personal experiences which have a meaning for their listeners.

The interview

Other interviews are recorded on a one to one basis where the researcher will visit the interviewee in his or her own home and record recollections on a particular theme, explaining that these stories may well find their way into one of Age

Exchange's theatre shows or publications. The response is usually one of excitement and surprise, since so many of the older people approached have very few occasions for talking at length, especially to an avid and enthusiastic listener.

Age Exchange is often working with very isolated people, whose old age is a time of disappointment and loneliness, when retaining a sense of their own worth and selfhood is particularly difficult. Reminiscence can be an opportunity for reviewing one's life, taking stock, and seeing a pattern to events which is reassuring. It also provides an opportunity to get back into contact with those parts of one's life when there was a greater sense of potency and to remember that one is still the same person.

For those who work as carers in health and social services, or as individuals looking after elderly relatives and friends, reminiscence can provide a valuable insight into the personality and wide range of experience of old people, who may otherwise appear to them now as needy and passive. The pleasure of remembering the past can be animating and fun for old and young.

Ethnic elders and reminiscence

London has such a wide range of experience and background in its pensioner population, and Age Exchange has tried to reflect that variety by publishing the recollections of different ethnic groups. In 1984, a project called 'A Place To Stay' resulted in a book and a show charting the childhood experience of ethnic elders in their home countries, their decision to leave and their expectations of Britain. They were asked to talk about their early days in this country, of making a new life here and settling down permanently. They also spoke of how it felt to grow old over here away from 'home'.

Out of the stories they told us came a show, a publication and a touring exhibition. All these featured mother tongues and English, with languages alternating in the show, and sitting side by side on the page in the publication. Interviewing was conducted in mother tongues because many of the elders did not speak much English. Their fascinating, and often very moving, stories would not have seen the light of day without this research, as the people interviewed were not the sort of people who would commit their memories to writing or feel particularly confident that their experience would be of interest to others.

Interviews based on trust

It was not always easy to arrange interviews with ethnic elders, even when the interviewer was a mother tongue speaker, since people were often worried about who would use the information and whether there would be questions about their right to be here and so on, so much reassurance and explanation was required. Interviewers were often people who were organising clubs for ethnic elders, who therefore knew the individuals concerned, and who were keen that their groups should have a more public voice. In many cases, the interviewers were the actors who were going to perform in the resulting show, and they were concerned to represent the old people they interviewed as accurately and sympathetically as possible.

The motivation of the interviewer has a great effect on the quality and depth of these individual or group reminiscence sessions. Where the interviewer needs to know answers in detail to certain areas of questioning because he or she will be representing this material in another form, such as a theatre show, the interest will be genuine and the interviewee will be more clear about why the questions are being asked. Often actors make good interviewers for this reason. They value detail and encourage the old people to dig deep in their memories to provide it. It is detail which gives clarity and quality to reminiscence, rather than the generalised statements about being 'poor but happy' which often pass as reminiscence but are rather a form of nostalgia telling us little of substance.

Key issues emerging from the interviews

Some key issues which emerged from these interviews, which were often wide-ranging and covered a great deal of the personal history of the interviewees, will now be outlined. I shall use the words of the elders themselves to illustrate these points wherever possible. Where their views were originally spoken in mother tongues, the translations have been provided by the interviewers.

1. Loneliness

Separation from families and from old friends on coming to Britain has often meant an isolated old age for Britain's ethnic elders.

Caribbean woman:
> We all have loneliness, but thinking of old people of the Caribbean, this loneliness is new to them. Old people welcome a visitor, and for that reason, back home we would always remember that Granny Margaret lives next door and it would aways be my duty to send my children over to see how she is getting on, and she welcomed them. Here nobody wants to know. Everybody is too busy looking after their own business and the elderly then remain on their own, until it forms a part of their life.

Italian man:
> Now I find it very hard to fill my days, I read the paper for a while. Then I go out, I sit in the park, look at the other elders and I think, I am like them now. Yes, if I could I would really like to change. In Italy, in a small village, everybody is very close to each other, even if they belong to different generations. We have a stronger feeling not only for family, but for our friends too!

Indian man:
> I do get lonely and that's the only time when I think of my family and I wish I was with them, but I try not to think too much you see. You can be happy and I condition my mind to be so.

Caribbean man:
> Sometimes I sit in the park and think about the thing that I dread most and that is loneliness. Being a bachelor with no relatives, that is a worry.

Polish woman:

I can't understand how a person of 80-odd is allowed to live alone, with just somebody going in once a week to shop for them or clean the house. I can't understand that. In Poland they're not as well off perhaps, but at least they don't live alone.

Indian man:

We are people of Eastern civilisation. We take care of our children, but here they don't take care of us in our old age, they don't even understand what our feelings are. It's the system, the culture. My greatest shock is that I have lost my children.

2. Language barriers

Many of the elders we interviewed had not managed to acquire enough knowledge of English to communicate easily. In the early years of their stay in Britain, they had not felt any great need to learn English, since they were working with people from their homeland. Now, in retirement, many of them had lost contact with the friends they used to converse with in the mother tongue.

Greek woman:

Oh, when I first came to England I found the language very difficult, but I was working with Greek people most of the time, so there was no real need for me to learn English. It's only been in the last ten years that I managed to learn any English. I was working in a factory with English and Indian women, so I had to pick up the words and try and make some sense out of them in order to communicate.

Indian man:

My biggest problem here has been language, I can't speak English but I do understand it. If someone swears I know straight away.

Chinese woman:

In 1975, my husband died and we were evicted from our flat. I lost my husband, and I had no English. Suddenly I felt life was very miserable. Before that, though my work was hard, I had never felt that miserable. I had to prepare my husband's funeral. An Englishman talked about cremation or what. I didn't understand a word of his. I only kept nodding. He told me to select a coffin for my husband and I picked one at £500. He told me it need not be too expensive and picked a £300 one for me instead.

Indian man:

I had a very good friend who died in January 1981. He was very helpful to me. Whenever I had any problems, I used to talk to him. So I miss him very much. He was younger than me, but he was a good adviser. Whenever I had a holiday, and he had some free time, we would decide to visit the seaside. All our friends would get together and sit in his big van and go off somewhere. Sometimes we'd see an Indian film at the Aldgate Plaza or in Southall. He was not only a friend, this man, he was just like my own brother to me.

3. A longing for 'home'

There was a strong sense that Britain was just 'a place to stay'. In fact this became the theme of the final song in the play, as well as its title. As memories of childhood become particularly sharp in the later years, the *mal du pays* experienced by ethnic elders becomes more acute as the home country is continually in mind.

Caribbean woman:
> We all came for four or five years, but the time went on so fast, we just didn't think, until we end up doing 25, 30 years instead of five. Now we're here to stay. Where people had sold out their little holdings, they didn't have anywhere to go back to. They remained here continually trying to work to see how much they could accumulate to go back and start setting themselves up again. But time run out, y'see. They're still here and without anything accumulated to go back. So it's much better for them to stay where they are. Some are really prepared to stay. Others are compelled to stay and they accept it. 'I have to stay – well, I must be satisfied.'

Caribbean man:
> If when I first came here I had five years good money in my hand, then I could have gone back; then I could have done something for my home country. But at this age all I have is my pension to live on. How can you go back?

Italian man:
> I have not been to Italy now for 17 years, and I miss it dreadfully: though if I have to say what exactly I do miss, I could not answer. I have no idea how I would find it now, and if it is at all changed. It must be, mustn't it?

Guyanese woman:
> What I miss most from my youth in Guyana is the way of life. I miss the freedom. I knew a lot of people back home, nice people, you know.

4. Rejection of change in the homeland

Many people expressed considerable regret about the way in which the homeland had changed. Those who had returned to their motherland to visit fondly remembered, and in some cases idealised, scenes of childhood and youth, had often been horrified by the alterations, whether caused by political upheaval or more gradual evolution. There had been a forlorn hope too that the home country would have retained its social mores and moral standards, so elders had been shocked to find there many of the same problems of social disintegration as in contemporary Britain.

Greek Cypriot woman:
> Life in Cyprus has changed, it's become worse than in England. They used to put England down, but I am afraid they've got worse. Before, a girl would never go out with a boy walking along the street, but now they do, and the mother sees and doesn't say anything. Now I would be happy to go back to Cyprus for a holiday, but to stay, no.

Chinese man:

At last, in 1977, I made up my mind to go over [to Singapore] and see the family. It had all changed. It was just like being a stranger. All the houses where I had been before as a child had all changed. It was all new flats, new roads and even new names. They did ask me to stay, but I have been here in Britain such a long time . . .

Guyanese man:

I've been back to Guyana four times in 24 years. If Guyana was the way it was when I left in 1960, I would have gone back, you know, taken my time. But not now. Everything has deteriorated as I see it. It's everything, everything, the running of the country, the problems, the economy; to me everything is gone. Many people there feel people like us are darned lucky to be out of it all, y'know, and that is true.

Greek Cypriot woman:

I returned to Cyprus just after the War of 1976. Things have changed. Everyone has moved away, I couldn't eat because of all the suffering. It's a tragedy what has happened to Cyprus.

Polish woman:

I went back to Poland twice in the sixties. I saw all my family, and my mother was still alive then. It's all right there, but I would never want to go back for good, not the sort of Poland that it is now. Ever since we arrived here we've had to send parcels, not only food but also medicines, clothing, etc. And it's still like that now, even worse. So I've never wanted to go back for good.

Guyanese woman:

Guyana is different now. I went home 11 years ago and it's not the British Guiana I used to know. I mean all the beauty has gone out of it. I planned to go home after retirement a few years ago. I kept ringing up me family and they say 'You better stay where you are the conditions here are terrible'. Now you know if you have a British Passport you got to have a visa to go home. You can't go home without it to Guyana now.

5. Alienation from children and grandchildren

Many ethnic elders feel that the move to Britain has robbed them of their children, especially where the children identify strongly with British culture and turn their backs on the motherland as represented by their parents. The normal separation of young people from their parents is much more painful where issues of language, race and culture are involved. The inevitable sense of rejection is exacerbated by the fact that ethnic elders are often emotionally dependent on their children because of the difficulties involved in establishing their own natural friendship groups over here.

Indian man:

My children went to school here. I wanted them to be doctors or engineers but they let me down. They have betrayed me since coming here. They didn't become doctors or engineers. But they ended up running away with white girls. My daughter is the only one who hasn't let me down. She got married to a boy in India in 1980. He works in a fruit factory. They often come to visit us.

Imagine the dreams I had when I bought my house, it was big enough for all of us but now there is only me and my wife left in the whole house. What upsets me even more, is that my sons are not happy either, because my daughters-in-law have run away and got married to someone else. My sons are left twiddling their thumbs. I had told them it would not work out, but why should they listen to me?

Chinese woman:

My grandchildren are growing up here in Britain and therefore know little Chinese. They cannot express themselves well in Chinese nor can they write in Chinese.

Caribbean woman:

What I see here and I can't come to it is this. Back home, a grandmother looked after her grandchildren and lived in the house. So when, if a grandmother took sick, the family is there to look after her. We don't have to send our grandmothers to homes. Grandchildren grow up to respect the grandmother, and anything that happens those children are there to help. You see they support one another.... Grandmother plays a vital role as protector of that family. Grandfathers have their own role to play too, but the grandmother she is the greatest. There is nothing like that here in England.

6. A strong commitment to maintaining cultural identity

Although language is often the most obvious barrier between ethnic elders and their grandchildren, many also expressed a very strong desire that their grandchildren should be kept in touch with the mother tongue and culture, so that they retain a clear and separate identity, one which the elders can share with them.

Indian woman:

My grandchildren speak both English and Punjabi. They have preserved the Indian way of life, and my grandsons still wear the turban, even though their schoolfriends tease them about it.

Indian woman:

My children were getting older and forgetting the language that they knew. They were becoming very Westernised and they were losing touch with my culture and they could hardly understand when I spoke to them, so my husband and I decided to take them to India.

When we got to India, we got VIP treatment.... Somehow my village looked smaller now, but never did I feel that I didn't belong here. My children didn't like it at first. They were very frank and forward and not at all like the other children, but eventually they settled down. I knew deep down, though, that they were lonesome for England. I think my daughter missed England the most because she had so much freedom there, but in India she spent most of the time with me and the other women.

But my purpose was to teach them Punjabi. Now I am very proud that both my children speak and write Punjabi fluently and they are in tune with both cultures equally well. It was a struggle on my part along with my husband. But when I look at our children, it all seems worthwhile.

7. The desire for an educational role

Elders see themselves having a positive role here as educators and cultural leaders. Age Exchange have recently been initiating projects where ethnic elders work with schoolchildren, exploring their memories and telling stories about their lives. In two cases, one Asian and one Caribbean, the children are helping the elders to assemble a Reminiscence Box of objects and pictures associated with their homeland, together with suggestions for activities related to these objects. The boxes will then be available for other ethnic elders groups and schoolchildren to use. White children are involved in this process, learning about the different cultural patterns of the ethnic group, with very positive results.

Chinese man:

If the younger children ask me about the old customs I will talk about it. . . . In school they are taught English and at home they talk Chinese. That is very important and how it should be. They are learning Mandarin in a Chinese class too, so they know their own culture.

8. A need to be with compatriots

Clubs where elderly people can meet abound in this country, and in many cases the British-born pensioners who go there are also having to make new circles of friends following retirement from work, widowhood or a move to a new home. However, many ethnic elders do not feel at home in these clubs and prefer to have a separate meeting place. Ethnic elders themselves often feel frozen out by the majority.

They need a secure base where a common language is spoken, religious rituals are observed, familiar food is available and similar memories can be shared (see Age Exchange, *Remedies and Recipes*, 1987).

The affirmative qualities of reminiscence as a group activity are strengthened where links are readily established and common ground is easily found. Many elders expressed a strong desire to be with people from their honmeland. Since many elders do not have the blessing of a large circle of friends they have known for many years in this country, such circles have to be created.

Caribbean man:

You see this luncheon place a black pensioners' club [a Black Club]? On the other side of the road is the real thing run by the government. Black people are not welcome there. It's too cliquey and they gossip. A lot of Caribbean people feel they are outsiders. They are tired of overcoming difficulties. Tired of trying. They have to come out of their shells, become more like themselves.

Chinese man:

We have got a Chinese club now where the old people are always invited to go for Chinese New Year or any big Chinese occasions to have tea and cakes and a big dinner. And this year they have started carrying the dragon through the streets in old Chinatown.

Indian man:

Now my health has gone. I am often unwell and my sons live far away from me. My life is rather boring and lonely, I am often unhappy. Sometimes I go to the Gurdwara [the Temple] and meet friends, but that is all.

Polish woman:

I tried to hold on to some of our traditions, our Christmas Eve supper particularly, when we break bread in the form of a host and share it out with all those present on Christmas Eve, followed by Midnight Mass. I go to church every Sunday but I go to the English church, it's too far to the nearest Polish church.

Caribbean woman:

We are short of places to meet. We want more of such places. Some people will want to be together with people of their own kind; some will prefer to be mixed. People will want to know they are welcome to visit these places. People shut themselves in and decide to stay in. Sometimes it's despondency.

Indian woman:

Most of the time we go to the Gurdwara . . . as we don't have a television, a radio or a telephone. We speak to the people there and we also eat there. I don't go anywhere but the Gurdwara and I am very content with that.

However, many elders expressed a desire to avoid creating and perpetuating ghettos for ethnic elders, while recognising the need for a safe place to go and talk confidently with compatriots. The desire to reach out to other elders was expressed as follows:

Caribbean man:

I like to mix, I like to know people. I wouldn't like to stay only in my own community. It's no use being a multiracial person and just be in a ghetto. I would be most unhappy if it was my people alone. I have all sorts of friends.

Indian man:

More should be done to get pensioners together and help them understand each other. We should not be a special case as Asians.

Indian woman:

I trust God completely. Indians, whites, blacks are all the same to me. There is only one creator you see. My neighbours are English and they are very good to us. If I ever need medicine, I usually show her the bottle and she understands what I mean.

Dramatising memories

In Age Exchange reminiscence plays, the issues emerging from the interviews are dramatised. Wherever possible, the elders' own words are used, often set to music in the idiom of the speaker's own country. Memories of the different contributors are intercut in a way which brings out the common ground and makes the experience widely accessible.

Scene from 'A Place To Stay'

This scene showed the housing difficulties facing immigrant families. In the scene, the actors, carrying suitcases, criss-crossed the stage individually in straight lines but not colliding, to an accompaniment of ringing bells and knocks on doors in an urgent rhythm produced on Caribbean and Indian instruments by the musician. As each actor arrived at the front of the stage, he or she addressed the audience directly, while the other actors remained still. Then the rhythm began again and the 'search for a home' continued. Here follows a short extract from the text:

Indian man: When I came from India, I stayed with a friend while I looked for a place to stay. I had a lot of difficulties finding a house because landlords wouldn't let to people with children.

Turkish woman: My husband lived in Stoke Newington and we all had to live in this one room in a house with eight other families. We had to queue up for everything from the toilet to cooking on the same cooker. Five of us in one room.

Indian woman: Three years after my husband came, I followed him. We rented two rooms. There was no water in that house, and no heaters. The rooms are like prison cells and the walls of the houses are so thin that if one talks too loudly, the next door neighbours can hear everything.

Caribbean man: I had the experience of living in one room which was like a box. It was eight feet by six feet. You see little mice running all over the little room. I had to do everything in that one room. I fell off the bed more times than I care to remember. One day I cooked a meal in that same room. I put the meal on the table and the whole table collapsed. I cried.

Indian man: I was going to leave my job because I couldn't find a house. A white guy who worked with me told me not to leave my job, and he found me a house.

Turkish man: Where I lived, all the houses looked the same. I used to leave my milk bottles outside the door as markers, so that when I came back I could find the house without difficulty. One day I left as usual for work with the milk bottles outside, but when I came back I couldn't see a house with any milk bottles. I couldn't find my house and just wandered the streets.

Response to dramatised memories

The play provoked a great deal of discussion wherever it was performed, and at the end of each performance the actors and audience would meet to talk about the memories evoked by the piece and the issues raised. Many white pensioners enjoyed hearing these stories and said that they had begun to think for the first time about how black pensioners feel about being here.

Other white pensioners felt that there was too much self-pity expressed, and that they too had experienced difficulties and overcome them. The common sentiment of, 'If they don't like it why don't they go home?' was expressed by some white pensioners, but the play itself went a long way towards answering that question and on the whole the effect was very positive, especially where it was watched by mixed audiences.

Jewish elders

More recently, Age Exchange Theatre has created a show about the Jewish East End, charting the journey of Jewish families from Eastern Europe to the East End of London, and out again to North West and North East London. A community which had once been exceptionally tightly knit within a few streets in East London was now so widely scattered that many of the contributors had little contact with others who remembered the same sort of childhood. Their main contact was with younger members of their own families who might well not share their enthusiasm for discussing their roots and humble backgrounds. They were thrilled to work on the Age Exchange project, recalling their childhood days which were often remembered through rose-tinted spectacles.

Where interviews were conducted in groups in Jewish Day Centres and old people's clubs run by synagogues, a more balanced view would emerge as people jogged each other's memories about the hardships they remembered their parents enduring. But however bad things might have been economically for the immigrant Jewish community in the East End, the sense of community was the prevailing feeling then and the enduring memory now. The nostalgia for that sense of shared hardships and hopes was what made the present difficult to bear, even though many of those interviewed were in excellent situations from a financial point of view.

The Jewish community is often held up as a model of how a minority can accept its responsibilities and care for its own elderly and infirm population. Certainly the excellent organisation and varied programme of activities in the Jewish Day Centres was impressive, and there was plenty of evidence of a continuing link with Yiddish culture as well as religious observance.

The book of the Jewish East End memories has not yet been published, but promises to give a clear new vision of a close knit minority group taking over an area of London which has served as home to countless minorities over the centuries.

Irish elders

The Irish community in London were the subject of Age Exchange's most recent investigation. Interviewers visited Irish pensioners' clubs and many individuals in their own homes to record their memories of childhood in Ireland and as adults 'over here'. Many of the issues raised with ethnic elders in the 'Place To Stay' project applied equally to 'Across The Irish Sea'. The sense of loss of 'home' was acute and there was a growing desire to re-establish links with family from home in their later years. Efforts to go back and settle in the old country had largely failed as the image of Ireland carried around by elderly Irish people over here was often found to bear little relation to the much changed reality. So many fondly remembered friends and family were no longer there, that it was really the land itself which was most mourned and desired. The play ended with these words:

> It's surprising when you sit down and relive your life. I'm 50 years here now but I still don't feel like an English woman. I've given strict instructions that I'm to be buried in Ireland, and I've enough money put by to take my body over there. If I sit in my living room at home, in my rocking chair, my thoughts go to Ireland, to the ground, the soil, the air, the hills . . . they don't change.

There were always tears at the end of these performances, but also great happiness that the experiences they knew so well were being celebrated on stage by professional actors and published in print for all to see.

Suggestions for positive change

1. A need for acceptance on both sides

Caribbean woman:
> It's much better for them to stay where they are. Some are really prepared to stay. Others are compelled to stay and they accept it. 'I have to stay – well, I must be satisfied.'

Caribbean man:
> We are here in Britain now, and I think you are categorically mistaken if you now want to go back. You can't go to a country that can do nothing for you. You must stay in the country where you have done something for the country, so that it may do back for you. If you make a mistake, you can't make it right by making another mistake. How can you go back? What are you going for?

Indian woman:
> I like England. The English people have been good to us. Otherwise I wouldn't have stayed this long, and now I don't feel so isolated because there are so many Indian people here. I feel England is unique with its National Health Service. I admire this organisation very much.

2. More effective communication

Greater efforts need to be made to explain existing entitlements and facilities to ethnic elders, especially those who do not speak English.

Indian man:
> I think England is the best place to grow old in because of facilities granted, but only but only if we know what we can get and what benefits we are entitled to.

3. Financial support for families maintaining elders

Caribbean woman:
> Give the people a home that all the family may live together and die together. How nice it is for an old person in her bed, with her grandchildren around her, and she die in peace with her grandchildren around her.

4. The need for meeting places

Ethnic elders need to have places to meet which take account of their religious and dietary observances, their language and their social needs.

Indian man:
> The government do not do anything for us Asians. They want us to become like English people, and join their Centres but the thing is there is a very big cultural difference.

Guyanan woman:
> Now I am back here – my church is here, they are very friendly. We meet often in groups and just the other day we were saying we should not forget each other outside the church, we should not pass each other in the street.

5. An educational role for ethnic elders

There should be encouragement for joint projects between young people and ethnic elders, so that cultural identity is maintained and greater understanding created.

Caribbean woman:
> I think a lot of young people are interested, and I think we could get them involved too, because whatever happens they'd be very good; they're strong, they have the energy to get around.

6. Encouragement for cultural projects

Reminiscence and life history projects (often incorporating music, dance and crafts) with ethnic elders are important and need support. It is valuable to record the lives of this important group of British citizens and to make their experience available to others both old and young. Meeting to create a record of their lives has proved a positive and life-affirming experience for the ethnic elders concerned and has improved self-concept and created new friendships.

Caribbean woman:

There's barriers between old and young, there's barriers between neighbours and neighbours, there's barriers between old and old. This country is full of barriers. This country is full of people who are in pain and longing. If we break down our own barriers, because we too can be isolated, then maybe we can help somebody else. . . . We have a future of using whatever we've got as long as we are here. Life is worth living. We can be cheerful.

7. Making resources available

It has been demonstrated that there is much interest and activity in the field of reminiscence with ethnic elders, and an urgent need for resources to make it more widely available.

A positive approach

Instead of ethnic elders and others regarding their presence here as a problem, a more positive approach is needed through cultural and educational activity. Our ethnic elders are an asset to our society if only we and they can see it that way.

Caribbean man:

We done a lot for Britain. We bring life to them, no matter what they say. They have, and we give them more. We give all our energy and our strength and all the riches that we can get. We give it to this country. We give them another culture and background that they didn't have before.

References

Age Exchange publications, all edited by Pam Schweitzer, are available from Age Exchange Reminiscence Centre, Blackheath Village, London SE3 9LA. Tel 081-318 9105

A Place to Stay: Memories of Pensioners from Many Lands.
Remedies and Recipes: Caribbean Reflections on Health and Diet.
Across the Irish Sea: Memories of Irish Pensioners.
From Stepney Green to Golders Green: a Tape of Jewish Memories.
Life Times: A Resource Pack of Reminiscences.

4

Meeting health needs by traditional medicine

Bernard W. K. Lau

Culture, medicine and ethnicity

Culture consists of all the beliefs, behaviours, and values that are useful and functional for a particular group. These are integrated into a logical system and handed down from generation to generation. It is an adaptive mechanism that provides the members of a cultural group with a system of vivid ideas that gives some coherence to the crucial events of birth, development, illness, and death, and solutions to life's problems that earlier members have found, by trial and error, to work. Naturally, the prevailing 'models', the cultural belief system of any society at any given time and place, dictate the nature of acceptable explanations. In some cultures, for example, illness is attributed to the activities of ghosts or spirits or of a living witch or sorcerer. As a corollary, it can be presumed that knowledge about disease and illness must necessarily fit into the general knowledge structure and belief systems of a society while pseudoappropriate explanations for altered physiological states may be a function of what is normal or expected within one's subcultural group.

It is now realised increasingly that culture is a determinant of the incidence of disease. This influence is exerted through the effects of culture on diet, occupation, lifestyles, health care habits, mating patterns and other psychosocial factors.

It has also been well recognised that culture does influence the manner in which a patient presents him or herself to the doctor. Basically people have strong desires or needs to make sense of how diseases are caused or spread, and frequently they classify illness within rubrics of the common lore of their culture. Whether a person allows symptoms to rise above the threshold of complaint depends on the ways in which that person perceives illness and is moved to act about it, as well as on relevant social relations and situations. Under certain circumstances, a symptom may be tolerated when its meaning is thought to be understood. The meaning of the specific symptom as perceived can be a key variable in the decision to seek help. Another variable is the patient's ideas about what causes illness. This may determine what kind of treatment is sought and whether there will be compliance with a suggested therapeutic regimen. As an example, chronic vague disorders or common childhood disorders may be assigned to folk treatment, while injury or severe illness with well-defined symptoms to 'scientific' treatment.

Thus, cultural influences operate at a number of levels and through various channels. Belief systems, modes of perception, and labelling practices, as well as the values attached to suffering and impairment, all influence the experience and expression of illness. All these beliefs and practices relating to health in any one culture are integrated into, and reflect the total cultural pattern of, that particular population. In effect, people learn to be ill in culturally sanctioned ways. The health problems that people perceive, the gravity imputed to certain symptoms or disease labels, how and where help is sought, are all affected. How one comprehends and responds to a bout of illness, accordingly, will be influenced by heterogeneities of culture associated with social class, ethnic background, education, occupation, and religious affiliation.

However, because social groups often have different gene pools, geographic environments, beliefs and customs, as well as resources and levels of technology, there is great variation in how they solve the problems related to the health and sickness of their members. Taking a step further, it would be a mistake to assume that people of different ethnic groups all have the same conceptions about what legitimately is to be brought to the doctor for help, and what should be done in response. Depending on their own particular ethnic heritage, the patients, more often than not, bring with them their own special values, beliefs, priorities and attitudes that may have developed over the years. Before a patient ever arrives to see a doctor, the cultural meaning of his or her symptoms, and the social implications of particular disorders, have already influenced the decision to seek medical aid. By the same token, it is equally erroneous to believe that people of different age groups will behave in the same way in the event of illness.

At this juncture, it is pertinent to note that a medical system is the pattern of social institutions and cultural traditions that evolves from deliberate behaviours to enhance health, whether or not the outcome of particular items of behaviour is ill health. Whereas medical systems emerge from human attempts to survive disease and surmount death, and from social responses to illness and the sick role, a medical system is undoubtedly an integral part of culture. Medical systems cannot be understood solely in terms of themselves; only when they are seen as parts of total cultural patterns can they be fully appreciated. Every culture has developed a system of medicine which bears an indissoluble and reciprocal relationship to the prevailing world.

What is scientific medicine?

Scientific medicine is the generic term for a specific mode of healing characterised by:

1. the assumption that all disease is materially generated by specific aetiological agents such as bacteria, viruses, parasites, genetic malformations, or internal chemical imbalances;
2. a passive patient role;
3. the use of invasive manipulation to restore and maintain the human organism at a statistically derived equilibrium point (health).

It has also been called variously 'orthodox medicine' (because it is presumed to have conformed to established doctrines), 'Western medicine' (since it originated and predominated in Occidental societies) and 'technological medicine' (for its extensive reliance on the non-human mediation of illness). The dominance of scientific medicine is assumed through its theoretical exposition, clinical elaboration, and technological advancement. Like Western science in general, it rests on scientific rationality; that is, all assumptions and hypotheses must be capable of being tested and verified, under objective, empirical and controlled conditions. However, this medical model is more plausible than practical.

When patients present in a doctor's surgery, their problems are often classified in Western diagnostic terms. More often than not, biomedical nosologies have little relevance for individual patients and their immediate kin, who typically assume responsibility for managing episodes of illness.

Since modern medicine requires a degree of emotional detachment from its practitioners, they tend to concentrate on the disease and avoid being distracted by their patients' unique personal feelings and experiences. Patients, therefore, are often isolated and treated as 'cases'. It becomes apparent that the orientation of Western biomedicine adopts an engineering or mechanical approach for repair of the human machine. Diseases are seen to arise as the result of 'mechanical' failures. In this context, Western medicine focuses on parts of the body, rather than on the whole body. Thus patients in the present system are more or less forced to surrender themselves to largely unknown doctors who will treat them completely independent of their social history. This kind of professionalism not only diminishes the doctor's capacity to respond empathically to culturally divergent patients, but also replaces experiential awareness with stereotypic judgments.

While health care professionals are trained to look on all patients as the same by virtue of visible physical similarities or operational diagnostic groupings, it is a deplorable fact that scientific medicine has provided no methodological space for the unusual, the peculiar, or the idiosyncratic. Worse still, in the immediacy of their desire to adapt modern technology, doctors may not be aware of the fact that large buildings, sizable staffs, and extensive treatment programmes do not necessarily make an adequate or effective health service. What they have forgotten is that for a healing system to be effective, treatment must be acceptable. Acceptability is a function of the attributes that users assign to the system. What has been ignored is the rather simple fact that the introduction of a health delivery system based on scientific rationalism is a major social change process that would certainly be subject to the same resistances that are true of other social changes.

Underlying social factors, and its potential for dispelling anxiety, fear and doubt, mean that traditional medicine may be more acceptable than modern medicine to some people. Traditional medicine aims to tackle primary cause while modern medicine is rapid and dramatic and tackles the manifestation of disease not cause.

What has gone wrong with scientific medicine?

Over the past decades, critics, both inside and outside the medical profession, have been casting around for an explanation for why scientific medicine, with all the advantages of modern technology, has failed to combat disease more effectively. It has become evident that modern medicine cannot cure all diseases and techno-logical medicine alone is not adequate for treating the startling variety of maladies to which human beings are subject. This failure of scientific medicine to find cures for the leading causes of death and disability, and its inability to deal with the consequences of chronic diseases or of emotional states, have nevertheless given impetus to the search for alternative treatments or parallel therapies.

The public has begun to realise that modern medicine is necessarily hospital-centred, yet the vast majority of medical problems do not require inpatient management. After all, scientific medical training is based around the hospital where the patients, presumably, are sick. In actual practice, the doctor rarely gets to see healthy people or find out what the circumstances are in which they best retain their health.

More importantly, in many Western hospitals the mainstay of treatment has become almost exclusively medications. These chemotherapeutic agents may be useful in altering the biochemistry and physiology underlying the medical conditions, but they often fail to address the full spectrum of causes that may be implicated in the aetiology, maintenance, and enhancement of the problem. At the same time, the increasing health hazards of taking modern drugs are now coming to light. A certain proportion of patients taking prescribed drugs are likely to suffer undesirable side effects of the drugs. Some of the drugs may also produce dependence; and complications due to interaction between the drugs a patient is concomitantly taking are just too well known. Nowadays iatrogenic disease is frequently cited as a reason for public disillusionment with medical advances. Many diagnostic procedures used in scientific medicine are no less risky as they are likely either to kill or to disable the patients by accident. In many cases morbidity and mortality may result simply from inappropriate use of technologies. Sometimes the expense and risks of the medical system are direct consequences of its increasing reliance on invasive procedures, technological gadgetry and potentially dangerous drugs.

In addition, the reliance solely on medication inevitably ignores the healing potential that can be elicited by a closer, more ritualised therapist-patient relationship in which there is extensive involvement with the patient, his or her family and environment. For similar reasons, such intrinsically powerful sources of placebo effects as touching, holding, chanting and specific behavioural commands are not accorded due consideration.

Recently there has been a growing uneasiness among the public that their health needs are not being met. They complain that Western-trained doctors are lacking in interest and understanding, are preoccupied with procedures, and are insensitive to the personal problems of patients and their families. Doctors have continued to treat physical symptoms with physical remedies, yet with progressively diminishing success. Indeed, the doctor who cannot empathise with his or her patients, and who speaks cryptically or tersely and does not provide adequate explanation, may be inviting them to seek reassurance elsewhere. In this respect, many doctors no doubt contribute unwittingly to some of their patients' decisions to turn to traditional healers, already established in some cultures.

It is clear, therefore, that modern medicine has shortcomings (other than mere lack of efficacy) which may have driven patients to seek out alternative practitioners. The increasing popularity of alternative, including traditional, medicine may then represent a 'flight from science driven by disillusioned patients critical of the widely publicised shortcomings of orthodox medicine'; 'an erosion of confidence in orthodox medical practice'; 'a failure of orthodox medicine to meet public expectations', or the fact that 'our patients turn to them because we are failing to meet their needs'. On the other hand, the practitioners of traditional medicine seem to meet at least the psychological needs of their patients better than the Western-trained doctors. This is especially true where modern medicine clashes with the cultural viewpoints of the patients. They may also be closely attuned to the health needs and aspirations of the people they serve and have come to identify with them who accept traditional or indigenous health beliefs and practices as cogent and commendable. Some of these practitioners even provide a family-orientated and intimate general practice, including such activities as making house calls.

Why then traditional medicine?

When a person is facing a serious problem there is a desire to know the cause of such an affliction. In response to this, many practitioners of traditional medicine are prepared to advise on a wide range of problems. In this regard, a successful practitioner is one who knows how to make use of his sensitive perception to discern his patient's problems, and who is skilful enough to provide his patient with a lucid and convincing explanation appropriate to the latter's cultural background, so that he can facilitate a decision at a time of difficulty.

Many of the patients who go to the practitioners of traditional medicine as well as to the Western-trained doctors, are perhaps more concerned about some under-lying social problem than the ostensible medical one. In reality, these practitioners do seem to be generally more sensitive to symbolic aspects of disease (i.e. illness). They are well poised to treat illness in general, and the personal and social problems to which it gives rise in particular. It has been observed time and again that many of these practitioners do have more insight than Western-trained doctors normally have into the underlying anxiety of patients about loss of physical integrity. They appear to be able to judge patients' anxieties and problems in historical and social contexts. They also seem remarkably skilled at eliciting patients' views of the nature and significance of their own problems. They are definitely better at giving meaning to the experience of illness and, through that and other means, producing a behavioural and experiential impact, whether or not they are able to change symptoms. In some instances, they will even go beyond the diagnosis and treatment of individual ailments, as they may use the occasion of illness to search for the presence of unresolved conflicts in the patient's social circle that may have caused the troubles or would impair recovery. Techniques of cure, in turn, may have the intended effect of reordering the social context – relatives may be enlisted in healing ceremonies and allegiances reaffirmed in a social catharsis. Sickness is made to signify the presence of underlying social disorder of which one person's symptoms are but the surface evidence.

As there are no sharp differences between patient's and healer's knowledge of, and labels for, parts of the body and categories of disease, practitioners of traditional medicine are regarded to share significant parts of their constituency's health beliefs. Their disease concepts and cure methods are developed from within the community and their explanations of disease are plausible to patients at their common level of understanding and experience. The message in folk-terms is concrete, compact, and familiar to the patient, and thus is easily understood and accepted. Also, the practitioners would not mind corroborating lay diagnosis, instead of attempting to produce unanticipated analyses of overt or hidden symptoms.

Illness, for some patients, is both an organic process – in which the focus may be on specific body parts and their relation to one another – and a social process in which illness is a metaphor explaining and supporting a larger universe of meanings. Therefore, even though the interpretation may at times be 'supernatural' and not 'rational' (from a modern scientific point of view), it is nevertheless meaningful and useful to the patient. Obviously, there may be psychological significance in citing a supernatural power as the cause of the patient's problem. Furthermore, these practitioners are far less neutral and emotionally detached from their patients, than are their Western-trained counterparts. Instead they will take a keen interest in each patient, not just as a body with a disease, but as a person with his or her own special identity. Much more time is spent with patients, especially in communicating with them. As a result, the healer-patient relationship is much more personal and concerned than the doctor-patient relationship. In the main, traditional healing systems, with their emphasis on the subjective experience of the patients and focus on the person rather than just the disease, have more closely approximated the ideal of 'holistic healing' than have modern professional systems of biomedical care. Traditional healers tend to offer patients and their families a more intimate and congenial relationship than most doctors and hospital staff are able to. Very frequently, they even take cues from the family about the 'desirable' diagnoses.

Contrary to common belief, accuracy of diagnosis and efficacy of treatment are in reality less important than the dispelling of anxiety, fear, and doubt – all of which may contribute to an illness by way of complicating symptoms and reactions. The fact remains that although the practitioner's pharmacopoeia and many of his physical techniques are not empirically effective in themselves, their utility is clearly enhanced when delivered in symbolic context. His touch by 'laying on of hands' may promote healing if it is imbued with a special symbolic value for the patient. At least, touching may have a significant psychological effect on many patients. In practice, the efficacy of a treatment depends largely upon 'whether the patient believes or not'. Usually the patient does believe, by virtue of the precision with which the practitioner fits theory and practice into the existing social structure and value system, and reflects the cultural and symbolic functions of the medical system of which he or she is part. In particular, the practitioner's ability in most instances to utilise the beliefs and ideas of the group as a fulcrum for influencing treatment increases the chances for the successful reintegration of the patient into the community.

Moreover, such practitioners often give people hope by treating the patient as someone who can be cured. They may insist that the patient has the capacity and, indeed, often the responsibility, to become and remain well. The prospect of help and a sense of hope not infrequently contribute directly to the patient's improvement. In this regard, many patients, particularly those with chronic problems which more orthodox medicine has failed to help, may find much comfort from these services. Indeed they may come to seek hope, if nothing else.

In all instances, the practitioner can exert a tremendous amount of personal influence and arouse a multitude of emotions in the patient, as well as in the group, during the course of a healing situation. This use of influence to arouse emotion may have therapeutic value.

The case of Chinese medicine as an example of traditional medicine

As part of the culture, the Chinese tend to value anything old and traditional. Such a tendency is reinforced by the belief that traditional medicine is effective 'gently' but 'radically', aiming to deal with the primary cause, while the effect of modern medicine is 'rapid' and 'dramatic', but it is merely tackling the manifestation of disease but not its cause. Such a view is supported by the less frequent occurrence of side-effects from herbal drugs in contrast to the seemingly more prominent side-effects accompanying modern medicine. In fortifying their arguments, herbal doctors always emphasise that the prescriptions have been transmitted secretly from ancient times and have survived an impressive test of time, enduring over millennia as the principal system of health care for a large population. No doubt the mysterious nature of such prescriptions proves to be very appealing to some people, particularly many patients suffering chronic illnesses who are looking for magical improvement. In some instances, the Chinese doctor deals with not only the patient's illness but also the patient's social reality.

In general Chinese medicine is perceived to be better than, or as good as, Western medicine in particular ways, such as for tonic care, for fewer side-effects, for curing the cause rather than merely the symptoms of diseases, and for treatment of certain diseases including measles, rheumatism, influenza and colds, bronchitis, anaemia, dysmenorrhoea, and sprains and fractures. Because it is chiefly concerned with function and the energy economy of the body, Chinese medicine has been said to be better equipped to deal with illness in its earliest stages, indeed, in stages so early that Western-trained doctors might not be able to detect them. It is believed by some that the most advanced organic illness in the world could have been cured when it was still functional.

For the purpose of representation, traditional Chinese medicine can be viewed as an holistic system in which health is understood as the co-operative functioning parts within a context. Health of the body is the microcosmic reflection of the harmony of heaven, representing a state of balance in the complementary and opposing forces of the universe. Disease begins as an imbalance in those forces, producing either excesses or deficiencies of basic life energy in particular organs or 'lack of ebb and flow' between yin and yang forces. If not corrected, these imbalances eventually produce physical changes in the material body. Treatment consists of manipulating energy flow around the body in order to draw excess energy away from organs with too much, and redirecting it to organs with too little. In other words, cure depends on restoration of the balance of elements.

The needs of elderly people

The illnesses of old people tend to occur in multiples rather than singly, and may be chronic or recurrent. They respond quite differently to medication and fit badly into categories. Response to treatment may be longer and physical recovery slower. Mental symptoms feature in physical disguises; social problems govern the response and outcome for the illness; textbook disease syndromes are the exception. In comparison to younger patients, although the medical problems with which old people are afflicted are no less amenable to treatment, the duration of an illness is usually longer. Treatment will need to be more prolonged, more specialised and is much more likely to be administered by a broad combination of disciplines rather than the core medical personnel; and the recovery from the illness is considerably slower. It is no wonder, therefore, that when older people become ill, they have special needs, different needs.

The greater prevalence of ill-health amongst elderly people naturally implies a more plentiful and direct experience of how modern medicine manages ill-health, which may in itself highlight the uncertainties surrounding medical interventions. This is understandable when it is acknowledged that the scientific perspective of modern medicine is usually more consonant with the intellectual orientation of the younger generation. As a result their faith in the value of modern medicine is by no means complete and they have considerable scepticism about the value of drugs. This is further reinforced by a set of attitudes (reluctance to perceive themselves as 'sick', less attention to symptoms, lack of information about treatment available) that makes them less likely to use the existing professional system in an active and purposeful manner. They would insist that not all health problems should warrant the intervention of a medical 'expert'.

This happens because elderly people have had many years to develop a sophisticated view of medicine that incorporates both public ideology about medicine and the commonsense knowledge gained through their own personal or private experience. Some of them may hold the view that modern medicine is good for critical conditions, but traditional medicine is essential to strengthen the constitution of people who are subject to frequent illness and should be more successful with functional illnesses. It is further surmised that modern medicine is good only for treating the symptoms and signs of disease, and they are looking for someone who will tackle that cause.

On deciding to seek aid, elderly people may be influenced by considerations of the conduct appropriate for members of the social group with which they wish to claim or demonstrate association. Those who wish to show how 'modern' they are may invariably consult a Western-trained doctor, while those asserting traditional values may look instead for a traditional healer.

In actual practice, elderly patients tend to use different methods of cure in a complementary and supplementary manner, as traditional and modern cures are often thought of as performing equivalent or complementary functions and supposed not to be mutually exclusive nor contradictory. On the other hand, traditional healers seem to be able to complement existing mainstream services and often refer people to the latter. So for many elderly the recourse to traditional medicine is not incompatible with conventional medical treatment. The sufferer, realising the ineffectiveness of such unorthodox endeavours, then returns to regular medicine.

Although it was true that traditional medicine was utilised primarily by the minority groups, there has been a more recent trend in the last decade that the majorities have begun to accept traditional medicine as a modality of treatment. This is particularly true in the case of the elderly. In fact, where mainstream health care is not readily available to this captive population, traditional medical practice will emerge to fill the gap.

As the practitioners of traditional medicine employ their own labour, the cost is significantly lower than that of conventional medical care. Moreover, for one reason or the other, it may be more personally satisfying to see the former than a Western-trained doctor. Apart from the reasons stated above, this can be accounted for in part by the fact that very little blame is placed upon patients themselves, and no significant responsibility for achieving self-improvement is given to them.

Conclusion

The nature of our industrial society is such that it produces large-scale institutions like modern medicine and inhibits growth of small-scale, low-technology, self-reliant groups. However, patients' and their acquaintances' experiences with modern care professionals and institutions have often been less than satisfactory. As a result, the desire for more personalised care and the greater availability of primary care has led to demands for traditional healers, who seem to be more friendly and down to earth, never talk down to their patients, have unlimited time, always offer an explanation the patient can understand, and always promise a cure. It is, therefore, not surprising that while the medical world awaits its reorganisation, traditional medicine starts to take up the slack.

The use of traditional medicine, for some, may reflect a general dissatisfaction with scientific medicine, or it may be used only for specific conditions and thus provide a complement to more conventional medical care. It has sometimes been suggested that modern and traditional cures can be made to complement existing mainstream services, while the use of the traditional healers rarely interferes with what a Western-trained doctor can offer. To this extent, dual systems should offer the most appropriate care. In some instances, the traditional medicine even provides the most successful treatment. Thus, patients can use different methods of cure in complementary and supplementary manner, to their advantage.

In view of this, there is a need for a solid understanding of traditional healing as an important aspect of the health care system and a central element in the education of health practitioners towards strategies for patient management.

5

Out of Africa:
a cross-cultural view of stroke

Simeon Onyejiako

In March, 1977, at the age of 44, I was laid flat by a stroke, and admitted to hospital in London. While I was there a doctor questioned me about my father's death – and this made me think back to my childhood and early life in Nigeria.

I was born in 1933 in a recognised experimental hospital in Cross River State, on the banks of the Calabar river – a river harbouring crocodiles, infested with mosquitoes, where mangroves intertwined with other plants and trees in the muddy waters. Although I was the only child of a polygamous family, we were poor because we had relatives and their children living with us and dependent on us. Most of the men worked as stevedores at the docks or wharfs, but the earnings were very small – only shillings a month.

Calabar was one of the oldest trading ports in West Africa. It created shanty township houses of small cubicled rooms, windowless and airless, housing large families. The staple diet consisted mainly of starch or carbohydrates, for example, yams, manioc or cassava, sweet potatoes, plantains, rice. For protein, we had goat meat, pig meat, bush meat such as deer, and – the cheapest food – fish from the fresh-water rivers and streams.

Calabar was notorious for supplying the cheapest alcohol to the population. There was a potent drink called *burukutu*, a fermented corn beer (a pint of this is equivalent to six whiskies). Burukutu and other alcoholic drinks were a menace to families, causing drunkenness, violence, and child abuse. Children suffered untold fear and anxieties, and because of malaria and other fevers they had heart conditions, boils and so on. I remember when I was five years old I had coughs, boils, fevers and jaundice, and a heart condition. Later, with the introduction of quinine, aspirins, and antibiotics, many children were freed from these troubles, but the insidious heart condition which began in my childhood remained with me until I was struck down with a stroke.

My education began at the Scottish Hope Waddle School, and continued at the Roman Catholic St Patrick's College, where I achieved London Matriculation certificate and a normal teaching practice certificate. One weekend, when I returned home from the College, I discovered that my father could neither walk nor talk nor understand us. He stopped eating, and we were very shocked. He lost his power of speech for a very long time. Our traditional herbalist was called in. The herbalists were called *Dibia*. Their herbal medicines were expected to have both magical and healing qualities. Some were foul-smelling and designed to drive away evil spirits.

Herbs were given to my father and he was advised to rest in bed. We knew the left limbs were weak and paralysed. The herbalist described the illness as *ogbubeng*, which is a word in *Efik* dialect; when translated into English, it literally means 'stroke'.

In 1950 my father was recovering and the wives and relatives were looking after him. There was nothing I could do for him and I decided to go to Lagos, the capital, in search of a teaching job. What I wanted to do was to study at the British Medical School, but I was told that medicine would be too expensive and too long a course, and that it would be better for me to study law – the course was shorter and, in the long term, cheaper. So what I wanted was a university degree. To this end I obtained a clerical job and worked in it five years. During this time I saved quite a lot of money and, with great support from my relatives, finally arrived at Hull University in 1956. But a year later my father died. That was a time of shock for me. It was my first mental anguish; I felt stranded abroad, and my savings were evaporating. I was depressed and anxious and could not concentrate at the Law School.

It seemed to me that this was the end of my academic dream, but my doctor sent me into the University sick bay where I was well treated, and eventually I joined the school again. In fact, in 1959, I was lucky to get a pass law degree, LL.B.

I then hitch-hiked to London, without much money, worked first as a kitchen porter and eventually as a school teacher in the East End, with a view to supporting myself until I was called to the bar. I met my present wife, Elsa, and we married within three months. Geoffrey was our first born in 1961, and looking after my family took me away from my continuing education. In 1965, our daughter Joy arrived and I was really struggling to keep my family.

In 1966 came the Biafran War, and I was very worried about the safety of my mother. I wanted to see her.

The war did not end until 1969 and it was not until September 1973 that I went to Imo State. I was lucky to find my mother still holding on in her ravaged village, but she was sick and haggard. So I decided to stay and look after her getting a job teaching English literature in Lagos. But the city was insanitary, violent and noisy. My salary was good but was paid infrequently. I began to fear for my health. So as my mother was better and I was able to leave her in safe hands, I returned to London in 1975 to look after my family.

There were many bills to be paid. I had to go back to teaching in Brent. This was my first experience with undisciplined pupils. They were quite unlike the Africans who were easy to manage and willing to study, because they knew this was the only way of personal advancement. This stressful teaching took its toll, and I decided to make a break and try to take a course in Child Development. This meant taking a year off from the school and going into a university.

At this time my blood pressure was very high. I began to have sharp pains in my left shoulder, to be panicky, sleepless and over-active. And eventually I went into hospital where I had the stroke.

The doctors and nurses were wonderful and gave me very good treatment. The loss of awareness of the affected limb, my sight, hearing and smell problems were looked into. In retrospect I think my speech was ignored and I was not sent to the speech therapy unit. I do not know why. I left the hospital after three months.

Recovery from stroke can be a long drawn out, tedious process. Some lucky patients quickly recover and suffer no permanent handicaps, but others are left with varying degrees of disability. Mine is basically speech and language difficulty. I can read and assimilate ideas but find it hard to explain things in words. At home I set to work to overcome this, using a collection of tapes, music, yoga drills, TV, and copying thousands of words from my library of books. I also read books and articles about stroke illness, including the CHSA publications. And I read about the experience of Roald Dahl and Valerie Eaton Griffith, who helped Patricia Neal to return to acting. But it was some years before I felt ready to apply to the Institute of Education to study Child Development, as I had planned earlier.

Taking this course was the greatest help for my speech and confidence. The foundation courses could have been designed for post-stroke people like me. It was good to have to write numerous essays and to keep rigorous timetables. There was a year's time limit for my course. With great mental and physical effort I finished my dissertation, had it typed and bound, and in 1985 I was awarded a 'Diploma on Adolescence in Nigeria'.

For a long time my wife and I had discussed the possibility of bringing my mother over to London. And in May, 1988, Elsa went to the remote village of Nsokpo in Imo State to fetch her.

Her visit was a great success. Of course, it was not possible for a 77 year old lady to adapt immediately to a very complex European city, but gradually we introduced her to public transport and departmental stores. We took her to buy clothes.

Food was easy. All sorts of foods are now imported into England. The staple foods of Nigeria are available all the year round – yam, farina, palm oil, stockfish, manioc or cassava. My mother loved everything I cooked for her.

By November, however, she was feeling cold and having arthritic pain in her knee, and she wanted to go home to see her house, her friends, her crops. So I took her home. On the way, we talked very often about *ogbubeng* or stroke. She agreed that both my father and grandfather had suffered in the way that I had in my illness. We talked, too, about the herbalists who practised the Igbo ethnomedicine culture.

Our welcome in Nsokpo village was hectic.

After a week I went to stay with Dr Cyril Nwanunobi, an anthropologist lecturer at the University of Nigeria. Here medical friends suggested that I should attend a lecture on ethnomedicine by Professor Anezi Okoro, a medical professor who had graduated in Edinburgh and London. This was the 1988 Ahiajoku lecture.

Igbo ethnomedicine has a history stretching back for 8 000 years, mainly based on knowledge of herbs and their curative properties. This has been intertwined with the folklore and culture of the people, so that cures have often been attributed to the warding off or vanquishing of evil spirits. But over the years, names have been given to many illnesses (including *ogbubeng* for stroke), and specific herbs have been used to treat these. The slave trade of the 18th century halted its progress. So many thousands of young people leaving the country had such a devastating effect that the herbs were no longer sought for and the knowledge of them was not recorded. But because so much wisdom and knowledge is always passed on by word of mouth, it never died.

The main theme of the lecture concerned the way in which Igbo ethnomedicine can be incorporated into modern medicare. Its greatest strength is in its knowledge of the medical use of herbs and plants, and it is believed that this can make a contribution to the pharmacognosy of the world. The World Health Organisation has recommended the incorporation of traditional ethnomedicine into national health programmes. But the lecturer expressed his belief that 'the most positive way to use traditional medicine practitioners is as a stop-gap while modern medicine spreads through primary health care to every nook and corner of the land. There is no way that a system that is severely restricted to *just offering herbal therapy* can adequately serve any community in this day of a comprehensive seven-stage modern medicare system.'

After hearing about my father's and grandfather's *ogbubeng* and their treatment, and thinking of my own experience in London, I believe I have a cross-cultural view of stroke. And I know that modern medicine saved my life.

Reprinted by kind permission of Mr Onyejiako and The Chest, Heart and Stroke Association who published the original article in the Summer 1990 edition of their magazine *HOPE*.

6

Walthamstow Asian elderly concern: an example of a self-help group

Durreshahwar Wassim

The immigration of Asian people to Waltham Forest dates back to the 1950s and 1960s and the current elders are therefore first generation migrants. The rapidly growing number of Asian elderly in Waltham Forest was of concern to their community. It was felt that little was being done to cope with their special needs and this was causing anxiety amongst the Asian community.

The tradition in Asian society is that the elderly person is looked after by a close relative or friend, but the different values and circumstances in Britain have caused significant changes. Asian elders were afraid that the bulk of the burden of looking after their needs would have to be met by the Social Services who were yet fully to come to terms with this section of the community who had different habits, customs, and culture.

Asian elders have considerable problems, for example loneliness, inappropriate knowledge of their culture by service providers, their religious and food requirements, cultural clash with their children and grandchildren, gradual disappearance of the caring atmosphere which normally existed in the extended family and shame at this loss of traditional care, difficulties in seeking help and assistance, concern at the availability of assessment of physical and mental health, difficulties with transport and language. One of the major problems is that Asian people by nature, irrespective of age or gender, will not relate problems unless confidence has been established and so an outsider asking members of the group what they require may find their questions fruitless.

Establishment of Walthamstow Asian Elderly Concern

A body was needed who could advise and stand up for the needs of Asian elders, as the local Age Concern had done for the indigenous elderly. The two groups now represent the elders of Waltham Forest between them and work successfully together.

The London Borough of Waltham Forest is on the London/Essex border and has a population of 215 000, 25 per cent of whom are from ethnic minorities. Of these 20 per cent are Asian. As with other minority groups, the Asian population has a young age structure with elderly Asians comprising only 5 per cent of the group, but as the total number of ethnic minority elders is expected to increase by 163 per cent by the year 2001, this change in age structure will present different issues to be addressed. In addition, although men will make up 54 per cent of the total elderly population, this will be 64 per cent in the Pakistani community, mainly due to wives being much younger. The numbers with severe disabilities is currently estimated at 3 per cent, but this will increase to 9 per cent in line with ageing, and will be 9 per cent of a larger total number.

Asian Elderly Concern in Waltham Forest was established in 1981 by a group of Asian people actively led by Mr Mahmood. The organisation has the following aims and objectives:

1. to promote the welfare of elderly Asians living in the Borough of Waltham Forest;

2. to develop welfare activities and projects for the benefit of senior citizens of the Asian community;

3. to liaise with the Social Service Department of the London Borough of Waltham Forest in the interests of Asian elderly.

As yet there is not a nationwide network of such groups for support and interchange of ideas, and not all minority populations have such a group working for them. The inclusion of this chapter in this book is intended to stimulate other populations to consider a similar development.

The London Borough of Waltham Forest provides some of the funding for Asian Elderly Concern, thus demonstrating its commitment to the organisation, and active fund raising activities provide the remaining income. The organisation has charitable status, is affiliated to appropriate groups in the borough and is represented at about a dozen meetings per month.

The group is directed mainly towards helping Asian elders, but will help any elder in need and, in accordance with the Equal Opportunity legislation, employ staff regardless of race.

The group is run by an annually elected management committee from the membership who promote the work and plan the welfare and social activities of the group. The social programme aims to address the problems of loneliness, disappointment, anxieties concerning illness and old age, and advice and explanation on the services available. The activities are planned to expand to particularly include elderly Asian women who have frequently led a secluded and lonely life and in many cases are much younger than their husbands and so feel more isolated when widowed.

Activities and services

Asian Elderly Concern aims to provide a cultural identity, bilingualism and Asian traditions with a firm religious base. Some of the particular activities are described below.

Luncheon club

This club was originally attended only by males. More recently, women have been encouraged to join but the male members retain a day solely for themselves. Women are able to socialise at the club and have prayers and other religious activities. The members highly acclaim the food and state that, 'It is indisputably one of the best luncheon clubs in the UK'.

Day centre

Members attending the luncheon club can attend earlier in the day to take part in recreational activities such as indoor games, Pakistani dramas and Indian films. There is also a reading room with Asian papers and magazines. A religious education class is available for elderly Asian women once a week.

Umrah trip

The Umrah trip organised by Asian Elderly Concern during 1988–9 enabled a group of 80 people to take part in a two-week tour to Mecca and Medina – the two most holy Islamic places in the world. An Umrah trip is the life ambition of every Muslim and the tour members considered themselves very fortunate to have attended. The Mayor of Waltham Forest was present at the departure.

Other trips

During 1990 a weekend trip to Paris, a day trip to Margate, and a day trip to Clacton were organised. The Paris trip included tours and a boat ride on the River Seine. These trips are very much enjoyed by members who are able to educate themselves about the holiday interests of other groups. Cultural activities are organised with the Asian Arts Council and three sight seeing trips were organised in 1989.

Hospital/home visits

Asian patients are visited regularly by officers and volunteers to ensure they get Halal food (if required), Asian newspapers and magazines, and other facilities. Housebound elderly are also visited and helped with meals and shopping.

Advice and counselling

Asian Elderly Concern offers advice on a wide range of issues, especially housing, pensions and benefits. There is a close working relationship with the Citizens Advice Bureau. Staff from the Health Authority and Social Services are invited to the Club to explain their work, answer questions and to learn about the needs of this section of their population.

Asian elderly home

Asian Elderly Concern in Waltham Forest is actively planning a ten-place sheltered unit in the borough, and already makes arrangements for accommodation for Asian elders with a local housing association.

Conference

In September 1990, Asian Elderly Concern held a seminar on 'The needs and provisions for ethnic minority elders'. This major event was organised with Age Concern, and was attended by the Mayor of Waltham Forest together with other officers from the authorities.

Conclusions

There are many perceived needs of the older Asian community and enormous work and resources are essential to provide the necessary services to meet those needs. Considerable initiatives are being taken and the aim is to further improve the services available to the local Asian elderly population.

7

Traditions of ethnic minority groups

Bashir Qureshi

A tradition is the handing down of beliefs or customs from one generation to another, especially without writing. Old habits die hard and it is no wonder that a patient's cultural or religious traditions influence the work of care staff. A cultural custom or religious belief has a long life and should never be ignored.

The aim of this chapter is to inform the care staff, planners and educators who are directly involved in rehabilitation about the traditions of some ethnic minority elderly patients in Britain. An overview of the most commonly observed traditions has been attempted as a first point of reference and the intention is to raise some issues in improving 'whole patient' care.

The rehabilitation team includes a general practitioner, consultant, hospital nurse, community or district nurse, physiotherapist, occupational therapist, speech therapist, chiropodist, dietician, pharmacist, social worker, patient and carer.

In 1948, when the National Health Service was formed, it was taught in medical schools and other professional schools that a health professional must practise 'patient care' without any regard to a patient's race, religion or creed (a set of beliefs or principles, e.g. culture). The intention was to avoid practising medicine with racial discrimination. It has now been clearly identified, however, that the issues of culture, race and religion are important influences on health and health care for all groups, and must be included in the education and practice of all relevant staff groups.

Religions

In modern Britain, most people follow six major religions and three non-religious persuasions. Three religions which originated in India are Hinduism, Buddhism, and Sikhism. Another three religions – Judaism, Christianity, and Islam – began in the Middle East. The non-religious persuasions common in Britain are Secularism, Agnosticism, and Atheism. Every religion has many sections and numerous sects. A person usually becomes more devoutly religious during an illness and also in convalescence or because of a disability.

Attitudes to religion

As a general rule, the ethnic majority do not mention their religion to strangers, even health professionals, because they consider it a very private matter and it is wiser to talk about the weather or holidays with such patients. On the other hand, almost all ethnic minorities, white or non-white, live by their religion and would like to talk about it. A health worker should not hesitate to ask an ethnic minority man or woman, 'What is your religion?' 'Is there anything you want to tell me about your religious duties and taboos?' Tables 7.1 and 7.2 show the main differences between religions, and the following examples indicate their influence on health care.

Table 7.1 Major religions: beliefs

Religion	God's name	Prophet/ founder	Holy book/ place of worship	Large sections	Original country	Three main countries
Judaism	Yahwah	Moses	Torah/ synagogue	Orthodox, Conservative, Liberal, Reform Jews	Canaan/ Jerusalem	Israel USA Britain
Christianity	God	Jesus Christ	Bible/ church	Catholicism, Protestantism, Eastern orthodox, Jehovah's witnesses	Bethlehem, near Jerusalem	Italy France Britain
Islam	Allah	Mohammed	Quran (arabic)/ Mosque	Sunni, Shia	Saudi Arabia (Mecca)	Saudi Arabia Iran Pakistan
Hinduism	Bhagawan (gods and goddesses)	Unknown (? Aryans)	Bhagwad Gita/ Temple	Shaivite, Vaishnavite, Durga pujari, Jainism	India	India
Sikhism	Sat Nam	Nanak	Guru Granth sahib/ Gurdawara	No sects	Punjab (India & Pakistan)	India (Punjab)
Buddhism	None	Buddha	Tipitaka Pali Canon/ Stupa or Pagoda	Malayana, Theravada	India (Behar)	Sri-Lanka Japan S.E.Asia
Atheism	None (nature)	Unknown	Philosophy (Rational morality)/ No worship place	Secularism, Humanism, Existentialism, Materialism, Agnosticism	Russia	USSR Britain USA

Elderly Muslims in hospital will wish to pray during five specified times of the day. The daily ward routine and the rehabilitation periods will need to accommodate this. Prayers are preceded by ritual washing and a small room will be required for privacy.

During the month of Ramadan, a Muslim eats only before sunrise and after sunset and fasts during the day. Fasting is excused during sickness, pregnancy and lactation.

Table 7.2 Major religions: customs

Religion	Calendar/ Holy day	Main festivals	Popular rituals	Religious foods	Taboo foods	Medical taboos
Judaism	Lunisolar/ Saturday	Sabbath, Yom Kippur, Passover	Kosher food, male circumcision, Bar/Bat mitzvah	Kosher bread, wine	Pork, shellfish, non-Kosher foods	Oral pork medicines, euthanasia, abortion
Christianity	Solar/ Sunday	Christmas, Easter, Pentecost, Lent	Christening, Holy communion, Confession	Bread (or com- munion wafers) and wine	Blood pudding (Jehovah's witnesses), Meat on Friday (Catholics) Alcohol (Legion of Mary)	Catholic taboos: abortion, contraception Jehovah's witnesses: blood transfusions
Islam	Lunar/ Friday	Ramadan, Eids, (two), Haj, Moharram	Halal meat, male circumcision, burial	Dried prunes, honey	Pork, alcohol, non-Halal meat	Pork and alcohol in medicine, euthanasia, contraception, abortion
Hinduism	Solilunar/ Saturday (or Tuesday)	Divali, Holi, Durga puja	Caste system (social class) Sacred thread ceremony, cremation, reincarnation	Laddo, ravri (sweets)	Meat (especially beef), alcohol	Beef in medicine or babies' milks, contraception, abortion
Sikhism	Solilunar/ none specific	Vaisakhi Guru Nanak birthday, Guru Gobind Singh's birthday	Khalsa symbols (uncut hair, comb, shorts, bangle, sword) cremation, reincarnation	Karah Parsad (sugar and flour)	Beef, alcohol, smoking	Beef or alcohol in medicine, contraception, abortion
Buddhism	Lunar/new quarter, Half, full moon	Vesakha (May), Kathina (October), Dhanima (Chakha day)	Paritta Sutta (protection sermon), Buddhist baptism, reincarnation	Milk and rice	Alcohol, intoxicants	Alcohol in medicine, contraception, abortion, euthanasia
Atheism	Solar/ none specific	Bank holidays, May day	Rational thinking and actions	Alcohol or soft drinks	Religious ritualistic foods	Anything against one's wishes

Customs affecting rehabilitation service

Interestingly, what may be acceptable in one religion might be forbidden in another and a health professional must be aware of some facts. Examples of these are given below.

Alcohol

Excessive use of alcohol is discouraged in all religions. Moderate use of alcohol, however, is permitted in Christianity and Judaism. Indeed, 'pubs' are an important part of the social structure in Western culture. Furthermore, wine is consumed in religious ceremonies such as 'holy communion' and 'sabbath' respectively,

On the other hand, alcohol is forbidden in Islam, Hinduism, Buddhism and Sikhism. Devoutly religious people will not accept it in medicine, even for external use.

Staff should be sensitive to both schools of thought and should ask the patient for his or her approval where a diet, medicine, cream or gel contains any form of alcohol.

'Do you drink?' is a question that can get a misleading answer. People in the West consider 'drink' to mean alcohol but to others it may imply non-alcoholic drinks such as tea or water. It is better to ask, 'Do you drink alcohol?'

Sex segregation

Sex segregation, even in places of worship, is practised in most religions, except Christianity. Hindu, Sikh and Buddhist women prefer to cover their heads with a scarf or sari. Jewish women wear a wig to cover their hair and Muslim women wear a veil to conceal their faces from men except their close relatives. Sex segregation is believed to strengthen the institutions of marriage and family life, the idea being that 'the less you know of others (men or women) the more you stick to one'. The Christian custom of courtship, as with common law marriage, is probably based on the principle of 'try before you buy'. The idea is again to strengthen marriage and family life. Whereas although elderly Christians prefer to socialise with the opposite sex in a mixed day centre there is still much natural segregation. Non-Westernised elderly ethnic minority patients will probably choose to go to separate rooms to meet their own sex in a day centre.

Food taboos

An occupational therapist may ask an elderly or disabled person to prepare a meal in a hospital or home kitchen. It is wise to remember food taboos in the patient's religion. Even if a patient agrees to cook a meal containing a forbidden meat, out of politeness or to please the occupational therapist, he or she may well suffer the agony of guilt feelings.

A short list of possible religious taboo foods should be remembered and it can be expanded in consultation with an individual patient. Some common food taboos are:

- all meat, animal fat and alcohol (vegetarians including Hindus);
- all meat, animal fat and dairy products – eggs, milk, butter, ghee, cheese and yoghourt (Vegans);
- beef and cow fat (non-vegetarian Hindus);
- beef, alcohol (Sikhs);
- alcohol (Buddhists);
- non-halal meat, pork and alcohol (Muslims);
- non-kosher foods, pork and shellfish (Jews);
- alcohol, tea, coffee, cocoa and cola (Mormons);
- meat on Fridays (some Roman Catholics).

Lack of familiarity with certain foods should also be borne in mind. For example, some English people do not like eating plain yoghourt, Asians are not keen on cheese, many British people do not like eating garlic whereas most Italians, Asians and French are very fond of it.

Cultural concepts of health and disease

Broadly speaking, there are two cultures in the world. One is the Western culture and the other, the Eastern culture. Furthermore, there are many subcultures with regional languages and local customs. Cultural concepts of health and illness will depend on the person, place and time. For example, an elderly Asian or African woman from a rural part of her country may have a very different concept of health and illness from that of an elderly Englishman coming from Oxford.

A white Anglo-Saxon protestant with liberal views will possibly think of health as 'physical, psychological and social well-being', and will have a 'biochemical model' as the concept of illness where a disease is understood to be an unhealthy condition caused by infection or diet or by faulty functioning of a bodily process.

On the other hand, an elderly ethnic minority person from an African, Asian, or Chinese culture under various religious influences may not hold the same concepts. Many eastern patients believe that health means 'having no illness', and that disease is:

- God's punishment for a mistake or sin committed by oneself, one's ancestors, or one's community in this life or in a previous life (if the patient believes in reincarnation), and it can be treated by prayers and animal sacrifices;
- a consequence of magic or a spell caused by an enemy, a relative or a neighbour, who has approached a practitioner of magic and spells, and it should be treated by a holy man who can counteract the spell by prayers, charms, threads or sacrifices;
- the result of the environment (or Satan's mischief), and the cure rests with God who uses doctors and other professionals as a 'means' for treatment.

It should not be taken for granted that every patient has the same concept of health and disease as the health worker. Where a patient comes from a culture other than that of the care worker, every effort should be made to understand that individual patient's concept of health and disease in the light of the above information. There may be other unexplored concepts which must be taken seriously.

There are many ethnic rituals practised the world over and a health professional should be considerate of a patient's rituals related to health if only in accepting that these will strengthen willpower, self-confidence and the hope of recovery because the person has great faith in them.

Some people from Eastern cultures (e.g. Gujarati Hindu women) have tattoos on the neck and arms with God's names so as to repel misfortunes, accidents and illnesses. The tribal custom of having ceremonial scars on the face of African people has similar connotations, as does the wearing of metal jewellery – now becoming a fashion culture. The ritual of male circumcision for health reasons is common among Jews, Muslims, and 80 per cent of Americans and Africans, including Christians. The use of traditional medicine before going to see a doctor is not an uncommon custom among ethnic minority elderly patients. Mutual openness and respect between the patient and the care staff is essential in multi-ethnic patient care.

Traditional carers of elderly and disabled people

Western model

Europeans follow a nuclear family system. A man, wife, and two children are the inner circle. Elderly people form the outer circle and they themselves want to remain independent, with personal privacy, until the very last day of their lives. Most choose to continue to live in their own home, receiving visits from relatives and friends. They may also be entitled to receive welfare services such as 'meals on wheels' at home. When this support is not possible, elderly individuals may choose to go into a home for the elderly. Many ethnic minority patients who are very Westernised or have no extended family in Britain will adopt this model of care. The myth of the existence of the extended family in minority cultures must be questioned and the situation established in each case.

Eastern model

Most Easterners, including people from South America, traditionally live in the extended family system. The elderly form the inner circle, and their many sons, daughters and grandchildren make the outer circle. The illness of one individual poses a crisis of varying degrees to all members of the extended family. An elderly person gains more respect and authority in the family hierarchy. Therefore the traditional carers are the young family members. Customarily, the patients are nursed by their daughters whereas their sons provide the cost of care. For some people a parent receiving 'meals on wheels' or living in an old people's home would be considered an insult because it reveals an apparent breakdown of the extended family system. In such circumstances the social services staff should liaise with a son or daughter when assessing an elderly person for health needs, including rehabilitation to establish the availability of help. Nothing is ideal in this world and ideal systems do not run for long; it is essential for care staff not to take the tradition of the 'extended family system' for granted because this system can only work if every member plays a part. In Britain, some ethnic minority elderly persons may not have this support and may be too proud or shy to reveal this to a health professional. A practice nurse should explore the real position when helping the general practitioner to screen those aged over 75 under the 1990 Contract.

Communist model

In countries from Eastern Europe such as Hungary, it is said that homelessness, unemployment and loneliness are capitalist words which do not exist in the true Socialist vocabulary or the communist dictionary. In such countries, an elderly person has to adopt one of the relatives or, where there are no descendants, an outsider as the next of kin who must be an employed or self-employed person. The elderly person has to give a room in his house to such a person who is obliged to become the carer for the rest of that elderly person's life. The carer pays all the bills including the repairs of the house (which is shared by the State) and expenses for medical care. After the death of such an elderly person, all the property and savings are transferred to the carer. Fair play is ensured by a solicitor, appointed by the State, who visits the elderly person periodically and sees the carer separately. Ethnic minority elderly people from Eastern Europe are expected to increase in numbers in Britain in the 1990s because of the fall of the Berlin wall along with the lifting of the iron curtain in 1990, and may bring with them these established systems or expectations.

A care worker should be aware of all three models of traditional care and find out from the patient and the relatives which model is being followed.

Life expectancy and social aspects

Life expectancy is increasing in the United Kingdom as is shown in Table 7.3. There are also more females than males in the 50s age group and twice as many females than males in the over 75s.

Table 7.3   Life expectancy in years

	1968	1978	1988
Males	68.5	70	72.2
Females	74.7	76.1	77.9

Source: Government Statistical Survey (1990)

The life expectancy of people living in developing countries varies, and in those who survive various accidents and infectious diseases it is comparable to the British figures. Infant mortality is the main influence on life expectancy (see Table 7.4). It is expected that the ethnic minority elderly in Britain will match the life expectancy of their indigenous counterparts. This longevity may be 'unexpected' and not planned for.

Immigrant populations may show a 'three generation' cultural classification. The elderly (those over 75) and upper middle-aged (over 65) will retain 75 per cent of their old cultural characteristics from their countries of origin and they will also acquire 25 per cent of new cultural characteristics from the British culture through adaptation. These are first generation migrants. A second group of this first generation are the people of working age (say, 21–65 years) who will show 50 per cent characteristics of the old culture and 50 per cent characteristics of the new (British) culture because of the influence of peers and colleagues at their places of work. However, the second generation (age 7–21 years) will present with 75 per cent of customs from British culture and 25 per cent of customs from their grandparents' culture. They were either born here or came to Britain at school age. They may have a 'two culture conflict' and may even become hostile to their own ethnic group because they feel more British than the native British people. Finally, the third generation of children under seven who are born here will have 90 per cent characteristics of British culture and only 10 per cent characteristics of their grandparents' culture. To most people roots are of some importance. In addition to

Table 7.4   Estimates of crude death rate, infant mortality rate and expectation of life at birth for selected countries (most recent data)

Country	Crude death rate (per 1 000 per year)	Infant mortality rate (per 1 000 live births)	Expectation of life at birth/years	
			males	females
Africa				
Egypt	10	110	52	54
Kenya	14	92	47	51
Sierra Leone	19	215	44	48
Malawi	25	130	41	44
America				
Bolivia	18	138	46	51
Brazil	9	82	58	61
Jamaica	6	16	63	67
USA	9	12	70	78
Asia				
Bangladesh	19	140	46	47
China	7	49	66	69
India	14	122	46	45
Japan	6	7	73	79
Sri Lanka	6	37	65	67
Europe				
England and Wales	12	12	70	76
Sweden	11	7	72	78
Yugoslavia	9	33	65	70
Oceania				
New Zealand	8	12	69	75
Papua New Guinea	16	111	50	50
USSR	10	28	64	74

(data from UN, 1981)

the 'three generation' culture classification, other variables such as gender and social class should also be considered. Women and unemployed individuals may feel more security in clinging to their parents' culture, and so on. This concept and other social traditions (such as non-words in Eastern languages, eating customs, toilet habits, asking of personal questions, keeping an open house, presents not being a bribe, doctor phobia among children and the elderly, cultural taboos, moral issues, and attitudes to social services) have been described more fully elsewhere (Qureshi, 1989).

Ethnic attitudes to old age

It is wrong to say that old age is revered in Eastern culture but not in the Western hemisphere. Contrary to this common belief, many elderly people hold positions of great power in both cultures even after retirement. 'Good' and 'bad' are relative terms and of little value in a transcultural comparison. Although attitudes to old age differ in both cultures, the goal remains the same, that is the welfare of their elderly people.

The Western approach is to encourage all citizens to look after themselves from childhood through to old age, as long as they live. In order to do so, everyone pays insurance contributions and taxes as an investment to guarantee a pension and social welfare services in old age. The Eastern attitude, however, is just the reverse. In the Asian subcontinent, for example, everyone looks after others – not only relatives but also friends or people speaking the same language (language or religious brotherhood). In so doing there is hardly any money left over from the carers' income to pay enough taxes to the State to cover a decent pension and some welfare services.

Each system has advantages and also disadvantages. Whether one adopts the Western approach of taking care of oneself or the Eastern approach of looking after others in every way including financially (even neglecting oneself) the outcome is the same. The aim in either case is to make the society one belongs to a happy and enriched circle. A health professional should check every patient's individual attitudes – as well as the attitudes of the relatives – towards old age, because this information will affect management.

Death and religious customs

The major religious and non-religious doctrines described in this chapter have a significant influence on their respective followers. A detailed description of each religion's prescribed rituals is beyond the scope of this chapter, although they are summarised in Tables 7.1 and 7.2. Since it is not possible for every health professional to learn enough about all religions or persuasions, it is essential to know what to do when a person is dying and what action to take when death has occurred.

The next of kin should be asked about the family convictions and religious customs. Many religious people may wish to ask a religious leader (e.g. a priest, pastor, rabbi, pandit, guru or imam) to be present at the bedside along with the patient's relatives, to read the appropriate holy book at the time of death.

When a patient has died in the presence of a care worker in a hospital or rehabilitation centre and the patient comes from a religion other than that of the care worker, in addition to the observation of sensitivity and privacy it is wise to:

- contact the next of kin and/or religious leader to ask what rituals should be observed;
- inform the doctor so that all legal obligations can be fulfilled;
- avoid touching the body if possible, and if it is not, to avoid telling the relatives in order to spare them further distress; devoutly religious people may not want someone from another religion to touch the body in case it disturbs the soul;
- ensure support for the family is available during the bereavement period.

Conclusion

Every country in the world has ethnic minorities and Britain has become enriched by the wealth of many cultures, religions and ethnic groups now contributing to its society. There is, however, a world of difference in their traditions, expectations and needs. This chapter has attempted to cover a vast subject in a little space so the information presented can represent the tip of an iceberg only. Much remains to be explored. A caregiver for elderly ethnic minority people, in a rehabilitation centre setting, should use this information as a starter. If approached with sensitivity, patients themselves may be the best sources of information relevant to their own care.

References

QURESHI, B. (1989) *Transcultural Medicine: Dealing with Patients from different Cultures*. Kluwer, Lancaster.
UNITED NATIONS (1981) *Demographic Yearbook*. UN, New York.

Further reading

DEPARTMENT OF HEALTH (1989) *General Practice in the National Health Service: The 1990 Contract*, p. 9. HMSO, London.
FRY, J., BROOKS, D., and McCOLL, I. (1984) *NHS Data Book*, pp. 259–67. Kluwer, Lancaster.
MARKUS, A. C., MURRAY PARK, C., TOMSON, P. and JOHNSTON, M. (1989) *Bereavement in Psychological Problems in General Practice*, pp. 265–75. Oxford Medical Publications, Oxford.

8

Patterns of health and disease in the elderly from minority ethnic groups

Paul McKeigue

Background

Sources

Information on the health of Britain's ethnic minorities is available from analyses of routinely collected data on mortality (Marmot *et al.*, 1984a), hospital admission rates (Donaldson and Taylor, 1983; Ebrahim *et al.*, 1987), and from some population surveys which have included substantial numbers of people from ethnic minorities. Althoug few studies of morbidity in the elderly are available (Blakemore, 1984), data on mortality and morbidity in middle age can be used to predict the likely patterns of health and disease of different groups in old age. Country of birth is a fairly reliable indicator of ethnicity in the elderly, but will become less reliable as the population ages and more of those born in Britain become 'old' (*see* Chapter 1).

Data on mortality by country of birth are available for the years around the 1971 Census but at this time only a very small proportion of the immigrant population had reached pensionable age. Data for the years around the 1981 Census will be more informative but at the time of writing national mortality rates by country of birth have still not been published. The Hospital Activity Analysis reporting system included a record of country of birth for each hospital admission and this made it possible to compare hospital discharge rates for different diagnoses and ethnic groups (Ebrahaim *et al.*, 1987). This reporting system has now been superseded by systems based on the Körner dataset (DHSS, 1982) which does not include any information about country of birth or ethnicity and no further studies of this kind can be conducted without setting up special reporting systems in advance. It is essential to compare activity with expected use to identify variations in take-up which may reflect inappropriate or inadequate information rather than a variation in need.

Health of migrants

In general people who migrate tend to be fitter than those who stay behind, and for this reason recent immigrants usually have lower mortality rates than with the host population. This 'healthy migrant' effect tends to wear off with time (Marmot *et al.*, 1984b) and the link between ethnicity and a high level of social deprivation and high death rate has been established and explains up to 80 per cent of the variation in standard mortality rates (NETRHA, 1990). In first generation migrants, patterns of health and morbidity tend to resemble the pattern in the countries of origin rather than the patterns in the host population. For instance, French and Italian immigrants to the United Kingdom have lower coronary heart disease (CHD) mortality than the national average for England and Wales, reflecting the lower coronary mortality rates in France and Italy (Marmot *et al.*, 1984a). The prevalence of chronic obstructive airway disease in the United Kingdom is one of the highest in the world: migrants from outside the British Isles have much lower mortality rates from this cause than the native population (Marmot *et al.*, 1984a).

Some of the contrasts in morbidity between ethnic minorities and the native British population are summarised in Table 8.1. Existing data on the patterns of health and disease of the three main groups originating outside Britain are outlined below. An additional feature, that of bone density variations, has yet to be fully researched however. Smith *et al.* (1990) report that in single photon absorptiometry tests on healthy American born subjects of different race and under 30 years of age, Black subjects had a bone density that was 8.3 per cent higher than that of White subjects, 9.6 per cent higher than that of Oriental subjects, and 23.6 per cent higher than that of South Asian subjects. Furthermore, bone density of the South Asians was equal to that found in 50–60 year old whites. The authors conclude that, if loss of bone mass with age proceeds at the same rate, osteoporotic fractures may occur at a much younger age in Oriental and South Asian people. Another study (Weinstein and Bell, 1988) has shown that the rate of bone formation in Black subjects was only 35 per cent of that in White subjects and, as the reduced rate also reduces the possibility of error in the cycle, it is suggested that the diminished rate may preserve the ageing skeleton. There are obvious implications for health promotion – especially concerning the prevention of osteoporosis – in the vulnerable groups, and considerable implications for service planners.

Table 8.1   A summary of contrasts in morbidity between ethnic minorities and the native British population

	Native British	Irish	South Asian	Afro-Caribbean
CHD	+ +	+ +	+ + +	+
Diabetes	+	+	+ + + +	+ +
Hypertension and stroke	+ +	+ +	+	+ + + +
Tuberculosis	+	+ +	+ + + +	+ +
Other respiratory disease	+	+ +	+	+
Cancer	+ +	+ +	+	+ +
Alcohol-related problems	+ +	+ + + +	+ + +	+

Health of the Irish

Compared with the native British population, the health of Irish men and women in Britain is generally poor. One indicator of this poor health status is the total death rate: in Irish-born men in 1971 this was 14 per cent higher than the national average (Marmot *et al.*, 1984a). Selection for fitness at migration may have been less stringent for the Irish than for other groups, since there are no controls on immigration from Ireland to Britain. Respiratory diseases and alcohol-related conditions account for some of the most serious health problems among the Irish in Britain.

Smoking and respiratory disease

The combination of heavy smoking, poor living conditions and a high prevalence of tuberculosis infection acquired in childhood is probably responsible for the high morbidity and mortality from respiratory disease in Irish immigrants. Death rates from tuberculosis in 1970–72 were more than twice as high in Irish-born men and women than in the native British population. In an analysis of data from the 1978 and 1980 General Household Surveys the prevalence of heavy smoking (20 or more cigarettes a day) was 23 per cent higher in Irish-born men than in the general population (Balarajan and Yuen, 1986). This is consistent with the excess mortality from cancers of the mouth, throat and lung among the Irish-born during 1970–72 (Marmot *et al.*, 1984a). During the same period mortality from obstructive airways disease was 39 per cent higher in Irish men and 58 per cent higher in Irish women than in the general population.

Alcoholism and other psychiatric problems

The General Household Surveys for 1978 and 1980 found a 31 per cent excess prevalence of heavy drinking in Irish-born men compared with the national average (Balarajan and Yuen, 1986). Rates of alcohol-related problems in the Irish exceed those in the native British population by a factor of three or more (McKeigue, 1989). Psychiatric hospital admission rates for alcoholism are five times higher in Irish-born men than in those born in the United Kingdom (Burke, 1976; Mather and Marjot, 1989). In a study at a general hospital in north London the admission rate for alcohol-related problems was three times higher in Irish-born than in British-born men (Taylor *et al.*, 1986). Mortality from alcohol-related causes such as cirrhosis of the liver, motor vehicle accidents, accidental drowning, homicide, and suicide is high in Irish men and women (Marmot *et al*, 1984a).

Morbidity in South Asians

With a few exceptions, the diverse groups originating from South Asia (the Indian subcontinent) share similar patterns of mortality and morbidity. These include high rates of diabetes and coronary heart disease and low rates of cancer. High morbidity from alcoholism is seen especially in Sikh men.

Cardiovascular disease

Death rates from coronary heart disease are about 50 per cent higher in South Asian men and women than in the native population (Donaldson and Taylor, 1983; McKeigue and Marmot, 1988). This high mortality is common to Gujarati Hindus, Punjabi Sikhs and Muslims from Pakistan and Bangladesh (McKeigue and

Marmot, 1988; Balarajan *et al.*, 1984). All social classes, from professionals to manual workers, are affected equally. Hospital admissions for heart attack are also higher than in the general population. The incidence of stroke is also high – comparable to that for the indigenous population (Smith and Jacobson, 1981). The usual risk factors for coronary heart disease – smoking, plasma cholesterol and blood pressure – are generally not higher in South Asians than in the general population. Although current guidelines on the prevention of coronary heart disease in the British population include a recommendation to reduce diatary intakes of saturated fat, there is no basis for extending this recommendation to South Asians at present. The only published surveys of the diet of South Asian adults are for Gujaratis in north-west London (McKeigue *et al.*, 1985; Miller *et al.*, 1988). In this group at least, dietary saturated intake is lower than the national average.

Diabetes

In the native British population the prevalence of non-insulin dependent diabetes in those aged over 40 is about 5 per cent (Forrest *et al.*, 1986). Prevalence in South Asians is about five times higher, reaching 30 per cent by the age of 65 (McKeigue *et al.*, 1988). As with the high coronary disease risk, this high prevalence of diabetes is shared by Hindus, Sikhs and Muslims alike (McKeigue and Marmot, 1988). A similar pattern is seen in other overseas South Asian communities and in urban India itself (McKeigue *et al.*, 1988). The risk of complications among South Asian diabetics is similar to that in European diabetics (Nicholl *et al.*, 1986). About one third of South Asian diabetics in middle age are undiagnosed, and this proportion may be higher in the elderly. Non-insulin dependent diabetes may be responsible for the sixfold excess of cataract operations among elderly South Asians compared with the native population, reported in a study of hospital admissions during 1979–83 in Nottingham (Ebrahim *et al.*, 1987).

The high rates of diabetes and coronary heart disease in South Asians probably result from an underlying disturbance of metabolism and body fat pattern (McKeigue *et al.*, 1989). The practical implications of this are that prevention of diabetes and coronary heart disease in elderly South Asians is likely to depend on controlling obesity. However this is unlikely to be a straightforward matter; in South Asian communities obesity is not necessarily seen as undesirable and may be considered a sign of health and social standing. The roots of this attitude lie in the association of poverty and low status with underweight in South Asia.

Smoking and respiratory disease in South Asians

Tuberculosis incidence is much higher in South Asians than in any other group in the United Kingdom: in adults the notification rate is 40 times higher in South Asians than in the native population (MRC, 1980). Separate data on incidence in the South Asian elderly are not available. Mortality of South Asians from this cause is five times higher than the national average. Smoking is common among Hindu and Muslim men, but only in Bangladeshi men are smoking rates higher than in the general population. The habit remains uncommon in Sikhs and in all groups of South Asian women. These low smoking rates are associated with low rates of chronic respiratory disease and lung cancer (Marmot *et al.*, 1984a).

Alcohol-related problems and other psychiatric problems in South Asians

Average alcohol consumption is relatively low in Gujarati Hindus, in Muslim groups, and in women in all South Asian communities. However heavy drinking and alcoholism occur in all groups including Muslims. Heavy drinking is commoner in Sikh men than in other South Asian groups but even in this group average alcohol consumption appears to be no higher than in the native population (McKeigue *et al.*, 1989). These consumption data contrast with psychiatric admission data indicating very high alcohol-related morbidity rates among men in South Asian communities where Sikhs predominate. In a recent study from a psychiatric hospital in Southall, all patients resident in Southall admitted between 1980 and 1987 with a primary alcohol-related diagnosis were ascertained (Mather and Marjot, 1989). Using 1981 Census data to estimate population denominators, the incidence of alcohol-related admission was calculated as 106 per 100 000 in South Asian men and 54.3 per 100 000 in European men. In women the rates were 5 per 100 000 in South Asians and 19 per 100 000 in Europeans. Other morbidity data are consistent with the clinical impression that serious alcohol problems are especially common among men in Sikh communities but indicate that Hindu and Muslim men living in the same areas are also affected.

The association between average alcohol consumption and the incidence of alcohol-related morbidity, though valid across other minority groups, appears therefore not to hold for Sikh men. One possible explanation is that Sikhs tend to drink spirits rather than beer or wine. This preference for heavy spirit drinking may be shared to some extent by Punjabi Hindus and may lead to more rapid dependence than the social drinking of beer and wine typical of native drinkers.

Cancer

Rates of the three most common fatal cancers – lung, bowel and breast – are lower in South Asians than in the native population (Marmot *et al.*, 1984a). Total cancer mortality in 1970– was 31 per cent lower in South Asian men and 10 per cent lower in South Asian women than in the general population. This low cancer mortality is shared by Hindus, Sikhs and Muslims (Balajaran *et al.*, 1984).

Morbidity in Afro-Caribbeans

The most serious health problem among middle aged and elderly Afro-Caribbeans is the excess risk of stroke and other conditions caused by high blood pressure (Marmot *et al.*, 1984a). Diabetes is probably also common in Afro-Caribbeans but the risk of coronary heart disease remains much lower than the national average, at least in Afro-Caribbean men.

Hypertension and stroke in Afro-Caribbeans

In national mortality data for 1970–72 mortality from stroke among Caribbean-born men and women was twice the average for England and Wales. Deaths attributed to hypertension as the underlying cause were five times more common in the Caribbean-born than in the general population (Marmot *et al.*, 1984a). Total mortality among Afro-Caribbean women was 30 per cent higher than the England

and Wales average in 1970–72 and most of this excess was attributable to strokes and hypertension. Similar differentials between Blacks and Whites in mortality from stroke have been recorded in the United States. This excess mortality from hypertensive disease and stroke constitutes a serious public health problem for Afro-Caribbeans in Britain. This high rate of hypertensive complications is not entirely explained by higher blood pressures in Afro-Caribbean men and women. Of three studies comparing blood pressure in Afro-Caribbeans and Europeans in the United Kingdom (Cruikshank *et al.*, 1985; Haines *et al.*, 1987; Meade *et al.*, 1978), only the study by Meade and his colleagues found higher blood pressures in the Afro-Caribbeans. The other studies failed to find a difference between the blood pressures of the two groups, but the number of Afro-Caribbeans in late middle age was small. It is probable that scene of the excess risk could be prevented by improved detection and treatment of high blood pressure in Afro-Caribbeans.

Diabetes in Afro-Caribbeans

Although no studies f the prevalence of diabetes in Afro-Caribbeans in the United Kingdom have been reported, there is a strong clinical impression that non-insulin-dependent diabetes is more common in this group than in the native population. Mortality attributed to diabetes mellitus was also four times higher in the Caribbean-born than in the general population. Evidence to support this comes from a study in Trinidad, in which the prevalence of diabetes in Africans aged 35–64 years was 12 per cent compared with 6 per cent in Europeans (Beckles *et al*, 1986). A similar difference in diabetes prevalence between Blacks and Whites has been reported in the United States (Harris *et al.*, 1987).

Smoking and respiratory disease

The high risk of stroke is balanced, at least in Afro-Caribbean men, by low rates of coronary heart disease and low chronic respiratory disease. The incidence of tuberculosis is three times higher than the national average in Afro-Caribbean adults. Smoking rates remain relatively low in Afro-Caribbeans (Balarajan and Yuen, 1986).

Alcoholism and other psychiatric problems

Data on alcohol consumption problems in Afro-Caribbeans are available from the General Household Survey (Balarajan and Yuen, 1986) and from surveys of blood pressure and cardiovascular risk factors (Balarajan and Yuen, 1986; Blakemore, 1986; Donaldson, 1986). These surveys are consistent in showing lower average alcohol consumption and lower rates of heavy drinking in Afro-Caribbean men and women than in the native British population. This low prevalence of heavy drinking is paralleled by low psychiatric morbidity for alcoholism among Afro-Caribbeans. In 1971 the crude admission rate in England and Wales for the diagnostic category 'alcoholism and alcoholic psychoses' was 14 per 100 000 in Caribbean-born men and 28 per 100 000 men born in England and Wales: for women the rates were 8 and 7 per 100 000 respectively. The total psychiatric admission rate, adjusted for age, was similar in the two groups (Cochrane, 1977). By 1981 the admission rates for both native-born and Caribbean-born men had risen by 75 per cent but the rates remained lower in Afro-Caribbeans (Cochrane and Bal, 1989). Similar findings were obtained in a smaller but more thorough study of psychiatric hospital admission rates in south-east England in 1976 (Dean *et al.*, 1981). Admission rates for other psychiatric diagnoses in Afro-Caribbeans were generally high, suggesting that the low admission rates for alcoholism in Afro-Caribbeans do not simply reflect a lack of contact with psychiatric services.

It has been suggested that racial discrimination is one of the possible causes of the increased rate of schizophrenia amongst Afro-Caribbeans, and that although assumed to be related to the migration process, recent work indicates that British-born Afro-Caribbeans have rates of diagnosis of schizophrenia higher than those of their migrant parents (NETRHA, 1990).

This has been shown to be up to 45 per 100,000 with those born between January and April running a 10% increased risk, compared with 10 per 100,000 for the indigenous population and 7 per 100,000 in the Caribbean. Murray et al (1991) has suggested this may be due to a winter virus, unknown in the Caribbean thus making mothers susceptible and detected in later life as mental illness.

Cancer

Total cancer mortality in 1970–72 was about 20 per cent lower than the national average in Afro-Caribbean men and women but the death rate from cancer of the prostate was more than twice as high in Afro-Caribbean men than in the general population (Marriot *et al.*, 1984a). Similar findings have been reported for Blacks in the United States. Although the number of deaths was low in 1970–72 this is of importance since prostatic cancer is common in elderly men, and the excess risk in Afro-Caribbean men may by now have become a serious problem in the elderly.

Health and social status

The data reviewed above have indicated that although morbidity from some conditions (such as diabetes and high blood pressure) is very high in South Asians and Afro-Caribbeans, this is balanced by the relatively low rates of conditions such as chronic respiratory disease and cancer compared to the native British population. The total level of morbidity, therefore, is likely to be similar in these groups to that in the native British population. Only in Irish immigrants is there a trend towards poor health in general. A survey of elderly South Asians in Leicester (Donaldson, 1986) suggested that levels of impairment in this group were similar to those in the general population in this age group.

Housing conditions and the extent of family support are important determinants of the need for health services for the elderly. In contrast to the pattern in the native British population, most elderly South Asians are cared for by their families. In the Leicester survey (Donaldson, 1986) more than 80 per cent of South Asians aged over 65 years were living in multi-generational households. For this reason, uptake of domiciliary services was low in elderly South Asians. The extended family is deeply rooted in South Asian societies and this pattern of family supports is likely to continue at least for the lifetime of most first-generation migrants from South Asia. In contrast, a survey in Birmingham (Blakemore, 1984) found that 40 per cent of the Afro-Caribbean elderly population were living alone. The need for domiciliary services in this group, therefore, is likely at least to equal that of the native British population.

Surveys of local populations will determine local needs, direct provision and indicate education and training of providers. The national picture should influence national education input and research findings will play an important part in planning and provision for changing needs.

References

BALARAJAN, R., ADELSTEIN, A. M., BULUSU, L. and SHUKLA, V. (1984). Patterns of mortality among migrants to England and Wales from the Indian subcontinent. *British Medical Journal*, 289: pp. 1185–7.

BALARAJAN, R. and YUEN, P. (1986). Health and social status of elderly Asians: a community survey. *British Medical Journal*, 293: pp. 1079–82.

BECKLES, G. L. A., MILLER, G. J., KIRKWOOD, B. R., ALEXIS, S. D., CARSON, D. C. and BYAM, N. T. A. (1986). High total and cardiovascular disease mortality in adults of Indian descent in Trinidad, unexplained by major coronary risk factors. *Lancet*, 1: pp. 1298–301.

BLAKEMORE, K. (1984). Health and illness among the elderly or minority ethnic groups living in Birmingham: some new findings. *Health Trends*, 14: pp. 69–72.

BURKE, A. W. (1976). Attempted suicide among the Irish-born population in Birmingham. *British Journal of Psychiatry*, 128: pp. 534–7.

COCHRANE, R. (1977). Mental illness in immigrants to England and Wales: an analysis of mental hospital admissions, 1971. *Social Psychiatry*, 12: p. 25.

COCHRANE, R. and BAL, S. (1989). Mental hospital admission rates of immigrants to England: a comparison of 1971 and 1981. *Social Psychiatry and Psychiatric Epidemiology*, 24: pp. 2–11.

CRUICKSHANK, J. K. (1985). Blood pressure and diabetes among West Indians in England compared with Jamaica. Unpublished MD Thesis, University of Birmingham.

CRUICKSHANK, J. K., JACKSON, S. H. D., BEEVERS, D. G., BANNAN, L. T., BEEVERS, M and STEWART, V. L. (1985(. Similarity of blood pressure in Blacks, Whites and Asians in England: the Birmingham Factory Study. *Journal of Hypertension*, 3: pp. 365–71.

DEAN, G., WALSH, D., DOWNING, H. and SHELLEY, E. (1981). First admissions of native-born and immigrants to psychiatric hospitals in South-East England 1976. *British Journal of Psychiatry*, 139: pp. 506–12.

DHSS (1982). *Steering Group on Health Service Information: First Report to the Secretary of State*. HMSO, London.

DONALDSON, L. J. (1986). Health and social status of elderly Asians: a community survey. *British Medical Journal*, 293: pp. 1079–82.

DONALDSON, L. J. and TAYLOR, J. B. (1983). Patterns of Asian and non-Asian morbidity in hospitals. *British Medical Journal*, 286: pp. 949–51.

EBRAHIM, S., SMITH, C. and GIGGS, J. (1987). Elderly immigrants: a disadvantaged group? *Age and Ageing*, 16: pp. 249–55.

FORREST, R. D., JACKSON, C. A. and YUDKIN, J. S. (1986). Glucose intolerance and hypertension in North London: the Islington Diabetes Survey. *Diabetic Medicine*, 3: pp. 338–42.

HAINES, A. P., BOOROFF, A., GOLDENBERG, E., MORGAN, P., SINGH, M. and WALLACE, P. (1987). Blood pressure, smoking, obesity and alcohol consumption in black and white patients in general practice. *Journal of Human Hypertension*, 1: pp. 39–46.

HARRIS, M. I., HADDEN, W. C., KNOWLER, W. C. and BENNETT, P. H. (1987). Prevalence of diabetes and impaired glucose tolerance and plasma glucose levels in US population aged 20–74 yr. *Diabetes*, **36**: pp. 523–34.

MARMOT, M. G., ADELSTEIN, A. M. and BULUSU, L. (1984a). Immigrant mortality in England and Wales 1970–78. *OPCS Studies of Medical and Population Subjects*, No. 47. HMSO, London.

MARMOT, M. G., ADELSTEIN, A. M and BULUSU, L. (1984b). Lessons from the study of immigrant mortality. *Lancet*, **1**: pp. 1455–8.

MATHER, H. M. and MARJOT, D. H. (1989). Alcohol-related admissions to a psychiatric hospital: a comparison of Asians and Europeans. *British Journal of Addiction*, **84**: pp. 327–9.

MCKEIGUE, P. M. (1989). Alcohol consumption and alcohol-related problems in the United Kingdom. Unpublished Report to Department of Health.

MCKEIGUE, P. M. and MARMOT, M. G. (1988). Mortality from coronary heart disease in Asian communities in London. *British Medical Journal*, **297**: p. 903.

MCKEIGUE, P. M., MARMOT, M. G., ADELSTEIN, A. M. *et al.* (1985). Diet and risk factors for coronary heart disease in Asians in North-West London. *Lancet*, **2**: pp. 1086–90.

MCKEIGUE, P. M., MARMOT, M. G., SYNDERCOMBE COURT, Y. D., COTTIER, D. E., RAHMAN, S. and RIEMERSMA, R. A. (1988). Diabetes, hyperinsulinaemia and coronary risk factors in Bangladeshis in East London. *British Heart Journal*, **60**: pp. 390–6.

MCKEIGUE, P. M., MILLER, G. J. and MARMOT, M. G. (1989). Coronary heart disease in South Asians overseas – a review. *Journal of Clinical Epidemiology*, **42**: pp. 597–609.

MEADE, T. W., BROZOVIC, M., CHAKRABARTI, R., HAINES, A. P., NORTH, W. R. S. and STIRLING, Y. (1978). Ethnic group comparisons of variables associated with ischaemic heart disease. *British Heart Journal*, **40**: 789–95.

MURRY, RM, JONES P, O'CALLAGHAN E. (1991). Foetal brain development in later Schizophrenia. In The Childhood environment & adult disease: CIBA Foundation Symposium 156. John Wiley, Chichester.

MILLER, G. J., KOTECHA, S., WILKINSON, W. H. *et al.* (1988). Dietary and other characteristics relevant for coronary heart disease in men of Indian, West Indian and European descent in London. *Atherosclerosis*, **70**: pp. 63–72.

MRC TUBERCULOSIS AND CHEST DISEASES UNIT (1980). National survey of tuberculosis notifications in England and Wakes 1978–79. *British Medical Journal*, **281**: pp. 895–8.

NETRHA (1990). *Health Services for People from Ethnic Minorities. A Report on a conference organised by North East Thames Regional Health Authority*. NETRHA, London.

NICHOLL, C. G., LEVY, J. C., MOHAN, V., RAO, P. V. and MATHER, H. M. (1986). Asian diabetes in Britain: a clinical profile. *Diabetic Medicine*, **3**: pp. 57–260.

SMITH, A. and JACOBSON, B. (1981). *The Nation's Health: A Strategy for the 1990s*. Kings Fund, London.

SMITH, E. M., COHEN, B. E. and WEINSTEIN, R. S. (1990). Racial Difference in Bone Density. *Journal of Bone and Mineral Metabolism*, **5**: Supplement S185.

TAYLOR, C. L., KILBANE, P., PASSMORE, N. and DAVIES, r. (1968). Prospective study of alcohol-related admissions in an inner-city related hospital. *Lancet*, **2**: pp. 265–8.

WEINSTEIN, R. S. and BELL, N. H. (1988). Diminished rates of bone formation in normal Black adults. *New England Journal of Medicine*, **319**: pp. 1698–701.

9

Communication

Deirdre M. Duncan

Communication is about people connecting, giving and receiving information and successfully conveying meaning by talking and listening, reading and writing and by gesture. Most important, its success is measured by the other person understanding and making sense of what is intended. Thus, underpinning it all, we must share a common channel for communication – shared words, gestures, or language. What happens where there is no communication, when meaning is not conveyed, there are no shared languages and no common channel? Then there will be frustration, confusion, possibly anger, and isolation. To avoid this negative situation, particularly with elderly people in a care giving context, we must set ourselves to develop channels of communication which are efficient and pragmatic.

This chapter aims, firstly, to set out the issues involved in communicating with the elderly from linguistic minority communities, and, secondly, to look at ways in which we can communicate more effectively in a care giving context with this elderly population.

Issues in communicating

Linguistic communities in the United Kingdom

One of the most fundamental challenges to our perceptions of British society today is the concept of multilingualism and multiculturalism. It is very difficult for many sections of our society to appreciate and understand the extent to which Britain is a nation rich in a variety of languages, religions, customs and cultures. Yet the opening chapters of this book make the case very clearly. It is for those in the caring and health professions to absorb this concept and to adjust their perceptions so that their staff and client management may reflect this greater awareness.

In the early 1980s, a study commissioned by the Department of Education and Science was completed and published as 'The Other Languages of England' (Linguistic Minorities Project, 1985). It drew a linguistic map, so to speak, of the country and sought to identify the range of languages spoken by the communities and where these communities were located. It showed that many large ethnic and linguistic minority communities live in the country's conurbations. However, social mobility and unemployment cause population shifts and there are many smaller linguistic minority communities throughout the United Kingdom.

There are implications for staff and client management from this study. Firstly, there should be continuous collection of demographic information in the district across several parameters, including ethnic and linguistic minority populations. Secondly, this information must be used positively to influence staff training and recruitment from these minority communities. In this way, resources may be in place whenever the need arises.

Clearly the number of linguistic minority clients will influence the amount of resources invested. Thus, it is important that there is thoughtful management to elicit the optimum benefit from constrained resources. For example, a health authority with a large Ukrainian or Italian or Vietnamese speaking population may be contacted for ideas and resource packages by districts with comparatively small numbers of these speakers. Further, human resources – such as trained interpreters – could be contracted to work across district boundaries or across disciplines in order to meet the needs of smaller linguistic minority communities. It is no longer possible to manage health care resources, in particular rehabilitation, without considering and planning for the management of ethnic and linguistic minority clients.

Ethnic versus linguistic minorities

'Ethnic minorities', a term used in this book, includes linguistic minorities. For the speech therapist and those interested in language and communication, it is important to appreciate the distinctions between the wider term and the subgroup.

The linguistic minority clients challenge, in a serious way, the communication systems used in the health and rehabilitation services. The language of the majority population is English – all staff speak it and for most of them it is their only language. Most clients' leaflets and letters are written in English, and most directions, signs and posters are in English. Yet many elderly people from linguistic minority communities have only a limited command of English, which is often context-dependent, for example greetings or language used in the workplace, while some have no English at all. They may have spent many years in Britain and never needed to learn English because their community satisfied all their communication needs, or circumstances prevented them from learning English. Such clients are monolingual in their home language, or possibly bilingual to a limited degree. There are also other elderly clients from linguistic minority communities who have developed both English and their home language and are effectively bilingual.

People from ethnic minority communities which are not linguistic minorities may have a dialect of English as their home language, such as Creole or London Jamaican. Dialect is a linguistic variation of a language, having its own grammatical rules, vocabulary and conversation rules. Dialect must not be confused with accent which is a regional variation of the sound system of a language, such as the West Country accent.

Both ethnic and linguistic minorities will have different cultural and religious axes from the majority English culture. Just as it is impossible to offer an acceptable stereotype of British culture, so equally it is impossible to offer an acceptable stereotype of other cultures, such as Punjabi, or Polish.

The implications for appreciating the relationship between minority clients and health staff in the rehabilitation services are far-reaching. A member of staff may be called upon to treat a client with whom he or she does not share a language nor culture nor many experiences. How do both start to communicate, to build up that all-important rapport, that relationship of trust, a channel of communication which will allow the health worker to pass on, and the client to take up the aims of his or her own rehabilitation? The remainder of the chapter will address these questions.

Naming systems

Our names are very important. Nothing is guaranteed to upset as much as our name being misspelt or mispronounced, or being given the wrong name or title. We choose a baby's name with care and we are usually careful not to express dislike for, or ridicule of, someone else's name. Names are often our first introduction to a person and exchanging names is the beginning of a relationship. Consequently, it is very important to make an effort to get names right and not to balk at names which we might find unusual. Names are our identity tags to our community and our traditions – not always, but often.

Naming systems throughout the world offer similar information about an individual – although they may do it in different ways which will be more meaningful to those within that society than to those outside it. An individual's name will yield information about the identity of the family or clan, gender, religion and class or caste.

Family/clan

In British and other societies the surname carries the family identity and is passed through the male line. Often at marriage the wife will change her name to her husband's, and the children will take their father's surname. Surnames become important identity tags in some societies but not so in other societies. In some countries where communities may live in small rural villages, there may be only two or three different family or clan names which lessens their importance and they may not be required officially. Hence, on coming to a country, such as Britain, which officially requires an individual to have a surname, some individuals might be unable to supply one, thereby throwing the first spanner in the works.

In some societies, the surname is passed through the female line. Also in some cases married women retain their family name in addition to their husband's although the children will only carry the father's name, for example Wong Fillmore (USA), Hernandez de Leon (Spain, Latin America). Finally, in some societies the family name will appear as the first name followed by the personal name, for example Mao Tse Tung.

Class/caste   Class or caste may be indicated by certain names. This is clearly illustrated in the Hindu naming system. Patel, for example, is a middle class name. In Britain, 'double barrelled' names (such as 'Hunter-Dunne') suggest upper class associations.

Religion

Religious names are given to indicate the individual's association with a particular religion. For example Mary or Joseph are associated with Christianity. In Sikhism, the religious name also carries the gender marker. Boys and men are called 'Singh' meaning 'lion' while girls and women are called 'Kaur' meaning 'princess'. It should appear as the middle name, enhancing the first name. However, if the family name is not used, it is often substituted for the surname. Hence, Mr Singh is married to Mrs Kaur. In Islam the names Mohammed, Allah and Ullah are religious names and should not be confused with the personal name; for example, Allah Ditta, Mohammed Ahram.

Gender

In many societies, personal names are segregated by gender. There are girls' names and boys' names, although it is not always clear cut. In English names such as Chris, Pat, Les, Sam and Billy are unisex. In Islam female personal names may be followed by Begum, Bibi, or Khatoon. In Sikhism personal names are not gender-bound, since it is the religious name which indicates gender. For example, Rajinder Singh is a boy's name and Rajinder Kaur is a girl's name.

Personal names

Many personal names include all the above characteristics – class/caste, religion and gender – and this is recognised by the members of the community. It is possible to identify common Muslim boys' and girls' names, Sikh names as well as Afro-Caribbean, Irish and French names, as well as those of other countries. Even more subtle distinctions can be noted, such as age, according to changing fashions. Compare 'Bill' and 'Wayne', 'Mavis' and 'Kerry'. One must be careful to avoid assuming too much. The name 'Thomas' is *not* Welsh but when it is coupled with 'Evans' or 'Jones' then the Welsh connotation is strengthened. There are also names which although broadly nationally identifiable, are not specifically linked to one community.

The meaningfulness of names within a society becomes more apparent with familiarity. The following names could spark off certain connotations in Britain, which may or may not be true: Fenella Horthing-Worsthrop, Elsie Sargeant, Michael O'Riordan, Donald McGregor. In Northern Ireland there will be associations made with the names William Brown and Eammon Joyce. In the same way, through familiarity, social meaning should be derived from the names: Sukjinder Kaur Dhillon, Noreen Bibi, Mohammed Yaqub Quraishi. Understanding a person's full name can be a powerful key to identifying the person and his or her traditions.

Some ethnic and linguistic minority people choose to call themselves and their children by English names; Balvinder becomes Barry, Giovanni becomes John. This choice may be an indication that they prefer to assimilate into the English-speaking society rather than maintain aspects of their minority language and culture. For a speech therapist this may suggest that, in the event of an acquired language disorder, pre-morbid language patterns may have been dominated by English.

The key to getting someone's name right is to ask them what they wish to be called and to let them know how you would like to be referred to. Learning about other people's names extends one's knowledge about people as well as about naming systems and the riches they contain. Understanding the elderly ethnic minority client's name is part of the basis of a good professional relationship.

Age

It should also be noted that some cultures follow the lunar calendar which adds 10 days per year to age thus adding one whole year every 36 years. Also some people from China and Korea calculate their age from conception, considering themselves nine months older than a birth certificate may state. Both situations can lead to considerable confusion.

Appropriate terms of address

Part of the process of establishing the basis of a relationship in rehabilitation with ethnic and linguistic minority clients is to develop appropriate terms of address.

Greetings

It is often the simplest things which are thought to be the most difficult to do. Learning to say 'hello' in a different language is one of those things. Yet it breaks the ice in such an effective and positive way that it is an important factor in establishing a relationship. Staff should acquaint themselves with manners of greeting in the language(s) of their clients. An English health professional or patient may either simply smile or say 'good morning' or 'good evening' once only to one person in a day and it is a way of establishing communication for the rest of that day. However, an Asian, Arab, African or Chinese patient may say these words (or their religious greetings) each time they see that person during the day. It could be as many as ten times because they are really wishing 'peace' upon that person and the more times it is said, the better. Westerners should not feel irritated by such an innocent custom. If individuals find this custom unacceptable, they should feel free to tell the person concerned that it is necessary to greet them only once a day.

Deference

In many communities, particularly religious ones such as Sikh, Muslim, Buddhist, the elderly members of the communities are highly respected. For women, notably in Muslim communities, it is only in their middle or old age or widowhood that they have the freedom to assert themselves and enjoy relative independence. In cases of educational or health decisions, it may be the grandmother of the family who will need to be consulted by the family and the professionals. It is important that the health professional recognises the status that some elderly people in ethnic minority communities enjoy. Deference and respect should influence their approach and management of this elderly population.

Appropriate questions

When obtaining case history information certain questions may obtain no response. For example in some Indian cultures it is not permitted for the wife to mention her husband's name. A woman in many cultures will not wish to discuss or give information about gynaecological matters to a male interviewer or even with men present. Persisting with such questions will have a very negative effect on rapport. Prior awareness of cultural sensitivities and customs, and working with a bilingual bicultural co-worker would avoid such gaffs.

The implications for using the appropriate terms of address is that a willingness is shown by the health worker to accept the elderly client's linguistic and cultural position. It is usually taken by the client and their family as a token of good will. As such it is a good beginning to the process of rehabilitation.

Facilitating communication

As a care giver or a member of the rehabilitation team, it is possible to facilitate communication with the elderly person from a linguistic minority community who has speech, language or communication problems, in the following ways.

Social grouping

In a situation where the clients are relatively mobile, they can be positioned and grouped with other clients from the same language group. This social grouping can facilitate and encourage communication among the group. Those with more English can perhaps communicate with the staff for those with less. This grouping should be altered during the course of the day for various reasons, but mainly to encourage social mixing which often deteriorates, understandably, with communication problems, and also to avoid ideas of segregation. There can be groupings for mealtimes, physical activities, occupational and creative activities, as well as groupings for language activities, videos, and so forth. In cases where there is only one member of a linguistic minority community, consideration should be given as to how best to integrate him or her into the group.

Communication aids

Recently, communication aids have become synonymous with high-tech gadgets. Communication aids can bring computerised speech and print to the non-verbal client at the press of a button. Aids to communication can also mean equipment which is much more low-tech.

The non-verbal client from a linguistic minority community may be able to benefit from a *communication board*. This is a non-linguistic method for communicating basic needs. It may be about twelve inches square and divided into smaller squares, each with a simple line drawing of the need or request, such as a cup meaning 'drink', a plate meaning 'food', a toilet, a telephone. It is recommended that care givers consult with the speech therapist involved before starting a communication board. In certain circumstances, where there are visual perception problems, a communication board would be contraindicated since the client would have problems using it. Further, with clients who are literate in languages which scan differently from English, that is right to left (e.g. Urdu) or base to top (e.g. Cantonese), some orientation work may be involved for them to benefit from visual materials.

Many elderly people use spectacles and false teeth and some may use a hearing aid. These are *prostheses* and are important to improving communication. Every effort should be made by care and rehabilitation staff to ensure that clients have these items easily to hand. It may even mean having two sets of the items – one for home and one for the centre.

In some cases where there is no bilingual co-worker or interpreter, the care and rehabilitation staff may wish to have some *basic 'emergency' vocabulary* with which to communicate at a minimal level with the patient. In such cases, it may be possible to identify certain key words or phrases, such as food, drink, pain, toilet/urine/bowels, yes, no. These could be learnt and understood by the staff in the appropriate languages or written out and put above the client's bed if necessary. Again the speech therapist would need to be consulted because in some cases the client's communication problem would prevent him or her from benefitting from this strategy. A further disadvantage to this communication strategy is that it is so minimal. It reduces communication between two people to less than a dozen words. In its favour however, it does offer some channel for communication of basic information and it is a strategy which can be built on. More vocabulary can be learnt as and when the need arises, for example 'medicine' or physiotherapist's instructions. More important, it shows both staff and patients/clients that 'a little goes a long way'. This limited beginning to learning and using a language shows a willingness on the part of the staff to meet the needs of their elderly linguistic minority clients. It is unrealistic to expect the elderly members of this population to learn English if they are not established bilinguals. The initial impetus must come from the staff and it will usually generate attempts from the patients to use English more successfully.

Communication is facilitated if the immediate environment is 'speaker-friendly', that is if the speakers and listeners or participants have some mutually interesting stimuli, such as culturally appropriate materials to work with, as well as pictures, posters, magazines, newspapers and videos in the mother tongue to look at. It is essential, particularly in long-term residential or day care centres, that the elderly clients from linguistic minorities can identify with their centre, even when several ethnic and linguistic groups are catered for. There should be some provisos made about literacy material. It is important to check with the client or their family that they are literate in their home language and/or English. In the case of a client with a language disorder the speech therapist should be consulted before offering them literacy material since they may find it frustrating and anxiety-provoking. Although they may be able to read the material themselves, linguistic minority elders may like someone to read to them. Local radio is often a source of information to the ethnic minority population. A radio programme 'Spectrum International' on Medium Wave 558/990 has been launched recently with programmes for Afro-Caribbean, Italian, Jewish, Asian, Chinese, Greek, Cypriot and Arab listeners in English and their own language. Some of the contributors to this book are guest speakers on health topics.

When there is no, or only limited, access to bilingual staff then encouraging volunteers from the linguistic minority communities to come to visit for a short while is an alternative. Care should be taken not to over-use or abuse the volunteer by demanding too much time or professional-type skills, such as assessment, counselling, interpreting in case-history taking. The volunteer's role should be to support the qualified staff in a designated activity so that the linguistic minority clients are encouraged to participate and socialise. These volunteers have a very positive effect on the socialising aspect of rehabilitation both within the centre and outside in the community. An interesting advantage to this strategy is that it may encourage more recruitment into the health service from the ethnic and linguistic minority communities.

Finally, when words fail there is always physical contact, such as holding a hand, patting a shoulder or giving a hug, which when used with discretion can be very effective.

Liaising with the family

It is most important for staff involved in the rehabilitation process to liaise with the client's family, to ensure that the nature of the client's problem and the concept and aims of rehabilitation are understood and that carry-over is happening. In the case of the client from the linguistic minority community, it is possible that these three objectives in liaison may take longer to achieve. It may be essential to involve a bilingual co-worker in this process, particularly in the early stages if the immediate relatives are not bilingual. Planning discharge from hospital and informing carers of the complex arrangements instituted requires much consideration and communication preferably in a form that can be referred to later.

Conclusion

It is important to appreciate the multicultural and multilingual nature of British society, and health care staff must reflect this in their communication with the elderly from linguistic minority communities. Some elderly clients will be bilingual but many will be effectively monolingual in their home language. Efforts must be made to become aware of cultural differences and thus to avoid offence or insensitivity to the elderly ethnic minority client. An understanding of names and using the appropriate terms of address will help to establish rapport. Several suggestions are discussed about facilitating communication, particularly with linguistic minority elders with acquired speech and language disorders, such as referring to the speech therapist, using communication boards and recruiting volunteers.

Further reading

LINGUISTIC MINORITIES PROJECT (1985). *The Other Languages of England*. Routledge, London.

Section II Health Care Professions with Regard to Ethnic Minority Elders

In this section, specialists look at their role, identifying and examining the salient issues in their particular field.

10

Ethnic elders and the general practitioner

Bashir Qureshi

Medicine is the science of medical knowledge, and general practice is the art of applying that knowledge to help patients and their families. General practice is the primary health care provided by a general practitioner (GP) to individuals and families who seek help by visiting a GP surgery near their homes and in the case of an acute illness or emergency, calling the doctor for a home visit. The GP is seen as an important member of the community by most people, and for people from ethnic minorities, he or she may be one of the only contacts with 'the system' apart from the religious leader. In the 1990s, the number of ethnic minority elders seeking their GP's help is likely to increase and all members of the primary care team should familiarise themselves with ethnic minority needs.

The 1990 contract

Under the 1990 Contract for General Practice in the National Health Service, all GPs must offer in writing an annual domiciliary consultation to patients aged 75 or over who are on their lists. Of course, patients are not obliged to agree, and retain their right to choose. A GP, on such a home visit, will assess the patient's sensory functions, mobility, mental state, physical condition including continence, social environment, and medication. The GP will record these findings in clinical notes and plan each patient's health needs. Unless inappropriate, depending on the elderly patient's state of mental health, he or she will discuss the plan with the patient. Two points in this contract will affect the care of ethnic minority elders: the one, that a GP is free to mention in the Family Health Services Authority (FHSA) local directories whether a link worker, who is an interpreter with multicultural knowledge, is available in the GP surgery; and the other, that a GP can also list in such local directories the languages spoken by his or her primary care team. In addition, any particular clinical interests of the doctor can also be mentioned such as 'there are provisions for providing appropriate care for the elderly with regard and respect to a patient's cultural, religious, and ethnic needs'.

The World Health Organisation (WHO)

The World Health Organisation has recommended the following criteria in providing primary health care (GP service) to all countries (Fry, 1983).

1. Primary health care should be accessible and acceptable to the people. It should be the nucleus of every system of health care and it must be well integrated into the system.
2. Primary health care has to be provided at a cost that the country can afford.
3. Primary health care must be understood by the public through health education and information.
4. Primary health care must be involved in care that is:
   - promotive;
   - preventive;
   - curative;
   - rehabilitative.
5. Those providing health care should include not only physicians but also other non-medical community health workers.

In the British National Health Service, under the New 1990 GP Contract, general practice will provide comprehensive patient care including:
   - promotion of health;
   - prevention of disease;
   - cure of disease (whenever possible);
   - relief and comfort (after an illness or in cases where cure is not possible).

Most of these criteria are already being met by many British GPs.

Size of ethnic minority group

An average GP in Britain has about 2 500 persons on his or her list. Nowadays no family doctor works alone or in isolation; each one becomes a member of a primary health care team which includes GPs, a practice manager, medical secretaries/receptionists, practice nurse, and attached community nurses (district nurses, health visitors, midwives). Among the attached community nurses there is almost always a health visitor for the elderly, and a psychiatric social worker. Some GPs either employ staff who come from different cultures and can speak various languages, or they may have Linkworkers – multi-ethnic/multi-lingual interpreter/patient advocates – available at their surgeries.

The number of a particular ethnic group will vary from practice to practice depending on the locality, the attitude of the practice's staff, and individual patients' choice. Although it is not possible to meet the needs of every ethnic group, a practical approach could be to identify a majority group in the practice, and the experience of identifying and meeting the needs in this way will pave the way towards appropriate care of all ethnic groups in the future. It has been suggested by Professor Jarman that the NHS and Community Care Act (1990) could disadvantage those patients considered to be 'expensive', including those from ethnic minorities (NETRHA, 1990).

Ethnic minority contact

John Fry (1983) observed that patients including the elderly from all ethnic groups consult their GPs for conditions, in order of frequency, as follows:

- **Specific minor conditions** (for example, acute throat infections, lacerations, dermatitis, ear wax, urinary tract infections, backache, vaginal discharge, vertigo, hernia and piles;

- **Chronic diseases** (e.g. hypertension, rheumatism (including osteoarthritis and rheumatoid arthritis), psychiatric illness including depression and dementia, ischaemic heart disease, congestive cardiac failure, obesity, anaemia, cancers, asthma, diabetes, varicose veins, peptic ulcers, thyroid disorders, parkinsonism, and chronic renal failure);

- **Major diseases** – the six most common are acute chest infections, severe depression, acute myocardial infarction, strokes, acute appendicitis, and cancers (lung, breast, gut, prostate, bladder, uterus and cervix).

Patients, particularly the elderly, from all ethnic groups consult their GP about social pathology (poverty, social security benefits, marriage, divorce, and crimes including assaults) and also seek advice on lifestyle matters such as smoking, drinking, overeating, undereating, and stress. As data quality improves the relationship between ethnicity and presenting condition can be determined thus facilitating prevention and response.

Ethnic minority patients, particularly those who are not westernised, will see a doctor from any ethnic group in an emergency especially when requiring surgical treatment including an operation e.g. acute abdomen due to appendicitis. However, for chronic conditions and minor ailments they are likely to try one or all of the following three approaches.

- **Conventional medicine** – they may see a doctor from their own culture, religion, race, and sex in order to avoid language barriers and cultural or religious conflicts.

- **Alternative medicine** – they may consult a practitioner of alternative medicine such as acupuncture (Chinese patients), Hakim's therapy (Muslim patients), Vaidic medicine (Hindu or Sikh patients), homoeopathy or health foods (all groups).

- **Self treatment** – many ethnic minority patients for various reasons will take advice from a friendly local pharmacist, a nurse living in the neighbourhood, another ethnic minority elder or health worker, and also from the rehabilitation care staff.

Registration and GP choice

Under the 1990 GP Contract, changing doctors has been made easier. The patient has simply to ask the doctor of choice to accept him or her on to that doctor's list. Since 1st April 1990, it is no longer necessary to approach either the Family Health

Services Authority (in England and Wales) or the Health Board (in Scotland) or the GP with whom the person was previously registered. GPs are also expected to issue practice leaflets to inform patients about the services and clinics they provide. Indeed, with the provision of more financial incentives in the 1990 GP Contract and a more humane approach to elderly people, it is hoped that the problems of registration and choosing a more caring GP will be resolved for elders from all ethnic groups. More ethnic minority elders are likely to wish to register with a GP who is sensitive to their language, cultural and ethnic needs.

Transcultural issues in elderly care

'Transcultural Medicine is the knowledge of medical and communication encounters between a doctor or health worker of one ethnic group and a patient of another. It embraces the physical, psychological, and social aspects of care as well as the scientific aspects of culture, religion, and ethnicity without getting involved in the politics of segregation and integration' (Qureshi, 1989).

A transcultural approach to medical problems, including those experienced by the elderly, may be useful in a cross-cultural contact during a medical consultation or health worker's course of treatment which may be as short as ten minutes or as long as one hour.

Let us examine transcultural aspects of some common medical problems that many GPs and rehabilitation care staff may encounter:

Rehabilitation and nutrition

Elderly patients, particularly those who live alone, are likely to develop a certain degree of undernourishment and malnutrition. However, the problem may be exaggerated by the avoidance of certain foods for religious or cultural reasons, which is not uncommon among ethnic minority elders in Britain. This subject is covered in more detail in Chapter 17.

Throat infections

Throat infections and chest infections are fairly common among the elderly. An English elder may be happy with a GP's reassurance or just a cough medicine. But an Asian may ask for an injection (or a course of injections) of antibiotics because of having more faith in the purity of medicine when it is given by injection. Reassurance is required.

Ear wax

The English or Scottish elders like to have their ears syringed by a practice nurse whenever they get wax in them. Ethnic minority elders may not be very keen to have this done. This may be because they are not aware that wax can lead to loss of hearing, and also because they are apprehensive about mechanical procedure (especially when it is carried out by a female nurse and not by a male doctor). One cannot but accept this innocent preference for the same sex because this custom is deep-rooted. Cultural habits die hard but these are in no way intended to upset people from other cultures. Of course, courtesy breeds courtesy. Sometimes a courteous chat can bring about a compromised solution to a cultural conflict.

Urinary tract infections

One of the causes of cystitis (urinary tract infection) in European women has been described as the wiping of the perineum with toilet paper, after defecation, forwards towards the urethra, because the infecting strain of *E.Coli* causing cystitis is similar to the ones found in the faeces. People from Eastern cultures hardly ever use toilet paper, even when living in Britain, and almost always wash the perineum with water after defecation. In this way cystitis from this cause is avoided. Moreover, as the female urethra is short and accessible to *E.Coli* from the perineum, particularly during sexual intercourse, it is likely that Continental women (e.g. French) who are accustomed to using toilet paper and then washing the genitalia and anal region in a bidet will have a lower incidence of cystitis from this source.

Urinary frequency and customs associated with excretion

A religious person may become more devout in old age. Urinary frequency can occur in uncontrolled diabetes, incontinence, enlarged prostate and also through the use of diuretics (for heart failure). A European male patient, when up and about, may pass urine in a urinal provided in a men's toilet at the same time as talking to another European man about the weather or current political issues. Because toilet paper is not provided alongside urinals, he may be content to dry his penis by shaking it about. The other man won't mind at all since he will be doing the same. Of course, they may use toilet paper at home. But all this will be abhorrent to an ethnic minority elder particularly if he is a Hindu, Buddhist, Sikh or Muslim. A person from one of these religions will prefer to sit in a closet and pass water. Speaking to another person during micturition is forbidden and it is customary to wash the genitalia after every act of micturition. Furthermore, being watched by another person, even a health professional, is stressful and worse still if the other person is from the opposite sex. In a rehabilitation centre the staff are predominantly female and may be unsure of the embarassment they may cause. Similarly an Easterner when in the toilet does not answer back if someone calls him or her from outside the closed door. He or she will make a throat-clearing noise in order to let the other person know that he or she is still in the toilet. An ethnic minority elder may even go home if he or she can, to use his or her own facilities. A man may be seen to take a milk bottle filled with water for cleansing when using a western style toilet. However, an eastern style toilet will have a low seat and a tap. Provision of a bidet will certainly help these patients. In addition to these embarrassments, ethnic minority elders with frequency of micturition or incontinence will be very worried about becoming unclean and therefore not being able to say prayers or conduct religious rituals. What may appear to be a trivial matter is in fact a crisis for some ethnic minority elders.

A health professional sensitive to the patient's needs and feelings can make life easier in three ways.

1. By talking to the patient and asking if there is any religious or cultural difficulty the patient is having. If so, what can be done about it?

2. By having a chat with the next of kin or a friend about the patient's needs in this context.
3. Through contacting, by phone or in person, the local appropriate religious leader for advice. In fact such a religious leader will visit the rehabilitation centre or any other place where the patient is and will not charge a fee. These religious leaders have a list of their followers, just as a GP has a list, and are a valuable source of help.

Prescribing drugs

The compliance with taking prescribed drugs will depend on their perceived value, as well as on their feared inclusion of alcohol or covering of gelatine capsule – either of which may be abhorrent to some individuals. These issues are covered in Chapter 17 and 18.

Surgical dressings and prayers

Some ethnic minority elders have to wash (the face, arms up to the elbows, and feet up to the ankles in the case of Muslims) or have a bath before saying prayers. A Muslim will say prayers five times a day, for example, and will have difficulty in washing if a dressing on his or her wound has to stay for a day or more. In these situations there are exemptions from religious rituals. For instance, a Muslim can use *tayamum* (role play of washing ritual without using water) because it is the intention that counts far more than the action in religious duties at the time of illness, travelling, or in unfavourable circumstances. Most patients will probably be aware of these allowances. Where this is not the case, a health professional should not hesitate to seek advice from the appropriate local religious leader and it is worth repeating that there is no fee to be paid for such advice. If medical or nursing advice is accompanied by religious advice, then the patient will accept it happily.

Ethnic disease patterns

Much literature is now available about some culture-bound illness which may be physical, psychological or social, and a further reading list is included at the end of this book. A detailed description of these diseases and an explanation as to why a condition is more common in a particular ethnic group is beyond the scope of this chapter. However, a brief mention of five diseases of the blood should serve as a stimulus for further reading.

1. Pernicious anaemia (Addison's anaemia)

Pernicious anaemia is a disease of the gastric mucosa. Sufferers often have recurrent soreness of the tongue and also prematurely grey hair. Pernicious anaemia is the most common cause of Vitamin B_{12} deficiency in the British white population and it is rare among Africans and Asians (Swash and Mason, 1984).

2. Sickle cell disease

A patient with sickle cell disease has haemoglobin S as a substitute for haemoglobin A in the red blood cells which become sickle-shaped. Sickle cells may obstruct the blood flow in nutrient vessels and cause infarction which may result in a sickle cell crisis. Sickle cell disease is most common among Africans, Caribbeans and Black Americans.

3. Thalassaemia

The common variety is Beta Thalassaemia, in which the production of Beta polypeptide chains of the globin is lacking. This blood disorder is most common in Greek Cypriots and Greeks but can also be found among Italians, Black people, Asians and South-East Asians.

4. Haemoglobinopathy D Punjab

This blood disorder is exclusively present among the Punjabis from Pakistan and India. Interestingly, Haemoglobin C disease is found mainly in Africans and Haemoglobin E disease is most common in South-East Asians (Indonesians, Malaysians, Filipinos and Chinese).

5. G6PD Deficiency

This inherited disorder is due to a sex-linked gene. The severe Glucose 6 Phosphate Dehydrogenase (G6PD) deficiency occurs particularly in Greek Cypriots and Greeks. A less severe variety occurs in some 10 per cent of African males (and less frequently in African females). This disease also occurs among Chinese and others from the Far East. Such patients do not have any symptoms but a haemolysis can occur after the treatment with drugs such as aspirin, sulphonamides, quinine, chloramphenicol, PAS, and after eating broad beans.

Conclusion

Cultural, religious and ethnic differences must be considered 'respectable entities' in science and should never be mistaken for 'inequalities' which is political jargon. To deliver an effective service, the composition of the practice population must be determined, together with the culture and language of patients. This will enable appropriate staff training and promote more effective care.

The importance of the role of non-medical care staff is being increasingly recognised by GPs who place more reliance now on the primary health care team when caring for elderly patients from all ethnic groups. The patient is acknowledged as the most important person in health care and the quality of care must be appropriate to an individual's needs. It cannot be overemphasised that medical, as well as transcultural, needs of patients must be met as skilfully and as sympathetically as possible.

References

FRY, J. (1983). *Present State and Future Needs in General Practice. pp. 1–43. Kluwer Academic Publishers (formerly MTP Press), Lancaster.*

NETRHA (1990). *Health Services for People from Ethnic Minorities.* Report of a Conference organised by North East Thames Regional Health Authority.

QURESHI, B. (1989). *Transcultural Medicine: Dealing with Patients from Different Cultures.* Kluwer Academic Press, Lancaster.

SWASH, M. and MASON, S. (1984). *Hutchinson's Clinical Methods,* 8th edn. p. 437. Baillière Tindall, Eastbourne.

WALSHE, J. (1989). *Dates and Meanings of Religious and Other Festivals.* p. 13. Foulsham Publishers, London.

11

The physician

James George and John Young

Britain is a multi-racial society. Elderly people of ethnic minorities are at a potential triple jeopardy: at risk through old age, through discrimination and through lack of access to health and social services (Norman, 1985). In order to provide good medical care doctors need to be aware of the background and special health problems and requirements of ethnic minority groups. This chapter looks at the requirements which may arise in the various departments of the hospital and at some of the specific medical problems which may be encountered by elderly people from ethnic minorities. Hospital services sometimes give a 'conveyor-belt' impression with patients being moved on from one area to another with little co-ordination. It is important at the outset to emphasise that care of the ethnic minority elder requires good teamwork and communication between departments. It is not satisfactory, for example, to provide an exemplary service in outpatients, with ready availability of interpreters, and then fail to follow this up if the patient needs to be admitted to the ward.

Outpatient consultations

It is essential to gain the confidence of the patient and relatives and this can be done only by taking an unhurried approach. Patience and a sympathetic attitude without condescension is required. In addition to the usual history, the following information will be helpful.

- The patient's country of origin: how long has he or she lived in Britain?
- The patient's religion.
- Details of languages spoken: the first language and any others.
- The extended family – how many adults and children are there in the household?
- Has the patient recently visited the country of origin? If so, when and for how long?

If there is a language difficulty it should be possible to use a qualified interpreter.

The question of country of origin and how long the person has been in Britain may be regarded as hostile by some people who do not wish to be questioned about their immigration status. This should be respected and the need to ask the question and its purpose fully explained.

Elderly ethnic minority patients may be particularly anxious and insecure, especially when it comes to examination in the outpatient department. Hindu, Muslim and Sikh women may be embarrassed at having to expose areas of their body to a male member of staff. Modesty should be maintained as far as possible and it may be necessary to arrange a return visit on a day when a woman can carry out the physical examination.

Casualty department

The Casualty Department is the 'shop window' of the hospital. Ideally it should only be for urgent treatment; non-urgent problems should be dealt with by the patient's own general practitioner. However, in many inner cities where ethnic minorities may predominate, there may be poor access to the GP outside normal working hours. Consequently the Casualty Department may be called upon. The Casualty Department should be sensitive to the needs of the local community. Interpreters should be available while signs and information sheets should be appropriately multi-lingual.

The introduction of health charges for visitors to Britain who have been here for less than six months does mean that patients may need to be questioned about their status. This should be done with tact and sensitivity, otherwise some migrants may be deterred from seeking much needed treatment, even though they may be entitled to receive it free. It is not necessary, for example, to demand to see a passport as a routine. The receptionist should be instructed in how to pronounce and record Asian names.

In a survey in the London Hospital, casualty officers found that 69 (12 per cent) of all patients seen in one week did not have a good command of English (Davidson *et al.*, 1983). Only 28 per cent of these patients attended with an outside 'interpreter', who was usually a friend or relative. The command of English of the outside interpreter was often little better than that of the patients. Communication problems can be major obstacles to delivery of health care, particularly in Casualty. A study in Birmingham showed that Asian patients with suspected myocardial infarction waited longer before being transferred to the Coronary Care Unit from Casualty because of language problems (Lawrence and Littler, 1985).

Caring for elderly ethnic minority patients in hospital

Communication

Many elderly ethnic minority patients will have only a rudimentary knowledge of English and the health care system and a qualified interpreter may often be needed. Doctors can help by being prepared to simplify their English and to speak slowly and distinctly. Non-verbal communication is important: for example, it is possible to reassure an anxious patient with a warm, welcoming smile, even if there is poor comprehension of the spoken word. Finally, it is always useful to check that they have been understood and to give written information, preferably in the appropriate language, to consolidate verbal information (Stevens and Fletcher, 1989). Such written information should be regularly updated.

Rehabilitation and teamwork

The concept of rehabilitation – restoration to normal function – may be a difficult concept to many people. Some elderly people from ethnic minority groups may not be familiar with disabling illnesses in which complete cure is unlikely, due to changes in life expectancy and other factors, and this will need to be explained. Teamwork is vital to good rehabilitation and it will be necessary to explain the function of the different team members and their importance as part of the rehabilitation team.

Cultural attitudes to medicine

To assist staff in understanding different expectations and beliefs, some relevant points are described for the main religions.

Muslim attitudes

In adversity, a Muslim is forbidden to despair and is required to be patient, seeking help through prayers. Older male Muslim patients are often unaccustomed to dealing with women with professional status and may sometimes be embarrassed with female staff.

In general a Muslim woman is not allowed to be examined or be surrounded by male members of medical staff and it is much more preferable if a female member of staff can be present. In some cases a Muslim woman may not agree to be examined by a male member of staff. Muslim women are normally required to cover their head and chest to maintain modesty and moral standards. Mixed wards should be avoided if possible and medical staff need to be aware of the requirement to maintain modesty.

Blood transfusions and transplants may only be accepted with reluctance by Muslim patients and will need full discussion.

Chinese attitudes

Western medicine has become established in Hong Kong and is accepted. However, traditional Chinese herbal remedies may also be used.

Chinese patients have no objections to blood transfusions or transplants.

Sikh attitudes

Sikh patients generally accept the authority of the professional, whether male or female. As with all Asian patients, women prefer to be examined by a female doctor.

Sikhs have no objections to blood transfusions or transplants.

The Sikh religion stresses an individual personal relationship with God and involves helping and serving others. Hence there is a strong tradition of action and community involvement amongst Sikhs which tends to make them seem more outgoing than other Asians.

All initiated Sikhs should wear the five signs of Sikhism – kesh (uncut hair); kangha (the comb); kara (the steel bangle); kirpan (a short sword); and kaccha (white shorts). In addition the turban has become a visible symbol for Sikh men and has similar religious importance as the five Ks. Sikhs in Britain differ in the strictness to which they adhere to the five Ks and turban. However, many will feel strongly that none should be removed and great offence and distress may be caused by unsympathetic understanding of these symbols.

Hindu attitudes

Hindu patients will generally willingly accept the authority of the professional. As with all Asian patients, a Hindu woman is likely to have a strong preference for a female doctor. Mixed wards should be avoided if possible.

Blood transfusions and transplants should not represent a problem.

Hinduism is the religion of over 80 per cent of the people of India. Hinduism has been evolving and changing over several thousand years. There is a strong sense of personal responsibility: actions and thoughts in present life determine the circumstances of the next. This is reflected in attitudes at times of crisis, such as illnesses which engender feelings of passivity and acceptance.

The family is central to Hindu life and obligation to family members is strong. Elderly people are revered and it is the duty of all younger members of the family to support and obey them.

Discharge and community care

Many of the ethnic minority elders are from inner city areas where there may be poor housing. They may not be receiving the appropriate housing and social benefits. Although ethnic minority elders are often supported by a close family network, this does not compensate for these other social disadvantages. A community survey in Leicester (Donaldson, 1986) showed that few elderly Asians were aware of Social Services such as meals-on-wheels, home helps and chiropody. Many potential problems can arise following discharge from hospital. For example, there can be a failure of communication between hospital and the community services and vital follow-up services can be omitted. Patients may overestimate their capabilities in hospital and experience unexpected difficulty at home. Also, sometimes patients may deteriorate at home because they allow their relatives to do too much for them, sacrificing their independence. These problems can occur with any group of elderly discharged patients but ethnic minority elders may be more at risk unless communication difficulties are overcome. Experienced liaison nurses can be invaluable in this respect, especially if they are familiar with the relevant cultures and religions.

Ethnic minority carers

There are more than one and a quarter million people in Britain who care for disabled or elderly people living in the community (Parker, 1985). The number of carers from ethnic minorities is unknown. Like other carers they need information and financial, emotional and practical support (Baxter, 1988). Access to information and benefits often depends on a person's ability to speak and read English, however, booklets such as 'Which Benefit' (FB2) are available in Urdu, Gujarati, Hindi, Punjabi, Bengali and Chinese, as well as English. Group support and respite care needs to be available for this group as for other carers. Much research still needs to be done on the particular difficulties of ethnic minority carers and how they can be helped with appropriate services (Baxter, 1988).

Medical aspects in care of the ethnic minority elder

Psychiatric illness

Psychiatric illness is difficult to diagnose in an elderly ethic minority patient and may go untreated. Stress due to recent migration may present in many ways, including anxiety, depression or also with somatic symptoms. A 'life change', such as moving to a new country, is likely to be particularly stressful if there is no social supportive network available, if there have been previous stress related problems and if the change is sudden and unprepared. For example, the stress on an English doctor and his family emigrating to Australia may not be very great, particularly if he has planned it for a year and has previously visited Australia and made friends there. Compare this with the stress on a 60 year old recently widowed woman who has spent her whole life in rural Southern India, and is suddenly taken away from her close friends to join her son in an English city. Not surprisingly, high levels of stress may present with predominantly somatic complaints.

Depression likewise may also be difficult to diagnose as the diagnosis is dependent on the history. Here, interviewing relatives and friends will be helpful. Likewise, the diagnosis of dementia is difficult as all mental function tests are based on language ability. Again, an interpreter and history from friends and relatives will be needed.

Transcultural psychiatry is becoming an accepted specialist branch of practice (Burke, 1989) and the psychogeriatrician needs to be aware of the influence of cultural factors in psychiatric assessment and treatment. This subject is further developed in Chapter 14, but the scope of this book is limited to physical rehabilitation, and another will be needed for the equally important subject of mental health.

Stroke

Risk factors for stroke are more common in some ethnic minority groups, for example hypertension in Afro-Caribbeans and diabetes in Asians, resulting in an increased frequency of stroke. Stroke illness makes demands at all levels of health and social service and also tests family relationships whatever the culture (George and Young, 1988). There may be misapprehension about stroke which may hamper recovery. For example, it is sometimes thought because a stroke is a sudden event then recovery likewise will occur suddenly, or that exercising the affected side is harmful and will prevent recovery. The modern concept of rehabilitation geared towards restoration of function will need to be explained. The patient and relatives will need to play an active part, otherwise recovery will be poor. A valuable member of the rehabilitation team is a social worker or health visitor with a special expertise in caring for ethic minority patients. A home visit may be necessary to ensure that the treatment package is realistic and that improvement is maintained after discharge.

Myocardial infarction

Myocardial infarction is roughly twice as common in Asian patients presenting to hospital but is only half as common in Afro-Caribbean patients compared to British rates (Hughes and Cruickshank, 1989). The extent of myocardial damage tends to be greater in Asians and coronary atheroma seems to occur prematurely and its progress is accelerated (Hughes *et al.*, 1989). Health promotion measures to prevent coronary heart disease needs to be directed at this group.

Hypertension

Hypertension is commoner in migrants from Caribbean countries leading to a higher incidence of stroke, but surprisingly there is a lower incidence of myocardial infarction (Cruickshank, 1989a). Treatment of hypertension in Afro-Caribbeans may need to be modified as beta-blockers and angiotensin converting enzyme inhibitors seem less effective (Cruickshank, 1989b). Apparent poor response to treatment may be due to racial variation rather than poor compliance.

Diabetes

Diabetes is more common in migrants from the Caribbean where it is predominantly a disease of middle age and early old age with a low frequency of early onset insulin dependent diabetes (Odugbesan *et al.*, 1988). It is frequently complicated by hypertension in Afro-Caribbeans in the United Kingdom, and it is important to take the blood pressure regularly in this group.

Similarly, diabetes is more common in Asians, especially non-insulin dependent diabetes. Diabetes is four times more common in Asian men than in white men and twice as high in Asian women compared to white women. Up to a third of these cases go undetected (Simmons *et al.*, 1989). It seems that Asian patients develop serious complications at an earlier stage than European diabetics and, therefore, need very careful follow-up (Nicholl *et al.*, 1986). Paradoxically Asian diabetic patients seem less likely to be regular attenders at hospital diabetic clinics. An innovative solution to this problem is to set up easily accessible local mini diabetic clinics run by a liaison nurse (Honey and Mather, 1987).

Osteomalacia

Osteomalacia or rickets is considerably more common in Asian patients. The reason for this is not completely clear but is probably due to a lack of sunlight, the consumption of chapatis, a diet low in vitamin D and genetic differences (Editorial, *British Medical Journal*, 1976). Osteomalacia is easily treatable with vitamin D and much more could be done to prevent this disease by giving appropriate dietary advice through Indian and Pakistani social and cultural associations (Editorial, *British Medical Journal*, 1976).

Diseases related to country of origin

It is well recognised that recent migrants from Asia and Africa have higher rates of tuberculosis than those who have been here longer (British Thoracic and Tuberculosis Association, 1975). Tuberculosis can present itself up to five years from time of arrival and may present as meningitis, bone and joint disease, lymph node disease or gastrointestinal disease rather than as pulmonary disease. Drug resistance (especially to isoniazid) may be imported. Spread of tuberculosis may be more likely because of poor and overcrowded housing conditions. Elderly people are more likely to develop side-effects with anti-tuberculous treatment. Physicians need to have a high index of suspicions for tuberculosis in recent migrants, particularly from India and Pakistan, and especially for non-pulmonary tuberculosis.

Other illnesses may occur when people from ethnic minorities revisit their country of origin, for example Asia, Africa or the Caribbean, and then re-enter Britain. Imported malaria is becoming an increasing problem and should always be suspected in somebody developing a fever on returning from a malarious zone. Diarrhoeal illness in returning travellers is common, often infective and may require hospital admission. Similarly, jaundice in a returning traveller may be due to hepatitis A, which is very common in developing countries. Hospital doctors need to be alert to these possibilities and should ask for details of international travel over the last five years. This question to the increasingly affluent and mobile younger generation may also be productive.

Case histories

Case study: Mr Qureshi

Mr Qureshi, an elderly Pakistani man, was admitted to hospital as an emergency following a stroke resulting in a right hemiplegia. His speech was unaffected and he had a moderate weakness of his right arm and leg. He had come from the Mirpur district of Pakistan in 1966, where he had worked on the land. He spoke Mirpuri and only a few words of English. His wife spoke no English. They were both devout Muslims. After three weeks in hospital he had made a good recovery, such that he could walk with an aid and dress himself. He was discharged home with outpatient follow-up.

One month later Mr Qureshi was admitted again because he had apparently deteriorated and become bedfast with his family having to feed him and wash him. In hospital he quickly became mobile and independent again and there was no evidence of a further stroke. However, when visited at home after discharge, he had again become bedfast despite his ability to walk. He was living entirely in one room with a commode, despite his ability to climb stairs and use the toilet. His wife was convinced he was a 'very sick man' and it was 'cruel' to ask him to walk. He gradually became more disabled and dependent.

Comment

It is well recognised that many stroke patients perform less well at home than in hospital, but in this case the degree of dependency was extreme. Mr Qureshi made a good functional recovery but he continued to perceive himself as disabled and ill.

This attitude was reinforced by his wife and family who wished to treat him as an invalid. Perhaps this situation could have been avoided if more attention had been given to educating the patient and family about stroke and the principles of rehabilitation. Effective use of an interpreter or a specialist social worker might have established a better foundation for recovery. A home visit, before the initial discharge (again with an interpreter), might also have helped.

Case study: Mr Ustinov

Mr Ustinov, an 84 year old Ukrainian man, was admitted as an emergency to a psychogeriatric assessment unit. The only history available from the general practitioner was that he had moved to a residential social services home three years previously following a left hemiplegia and subsequent inability to cope at home. The reason for admission was that over the previous week he had become very aggressive and abusive to the staff and the home felt that they could no longer look after him.

In hospital Mr Ustinov was found to have a chest infection which was treated successfully. His comprehension of English seemed good, although his speech was difficult to understand because of dysarthria. He had only a mild weakness of his left arm and leg but his standing balance was very poor. He needed two people to transfer him. He failed to improve with rehabilitation and was transferred to a continuing care geriatric ward. On the continuing care geriatric ward he was befriended by the nursing staff who were able to trace his background. He had been forced to leave the Ukraine and had been conscripted in the German Army. Following the war he had been sent by the Americans to Rome where he had made his way to England. His religion was Orthodox and he enjoyed his Ukrainian newspaper, sent to him by friends. He had been forced to leave his wife and children behind him in the Ukraine. He very much enjoyed talking about his experiences and showed no evidence of the aggression which had caused his admission to hospital. He was put in contact with the Orthodox Church and the subscription to his Ukrainian newspaper was continued.

Comment

Mr Ustinov's initial presentation was due to an acute confusional state due to a chest infection. Because of his poor English it may be that the correct diagnosis was delayed and his aggression was thought to be due to a primarily psychiatric disorder. Furthermore, perhaps if he had received rehabilitation earlier for his left hemiplegia, continuing care in hospital might have been avoided. However, Mr Ustinov settled in the continuing care unit very well and showed no signs of a behaviour disturbance. This may have been because the dedicated nursing staff paid considerable attention to finding out his previous history in order to make sure his needs were met. When his background was realised, he gained a new self-respect and it was possible to improve his quality of life by catering better for his religious and social needs. He subsequently became very interested in the news of the developments in Russia.

Case study: Mr Acharya

Mr Acharya, a 65 year old Indian man, was admitted to hospital with chest and abdominal pain. He had originally come to England from the state of Gujarat and he could speak Gujarati and Hindi but little English. Initially the diagnosis was unclear. He found it difficult to describe the pain or localise it. Subsequent investigations revealed that he had had a myocardial infarction and he was also found to have diabetes which was controlled by diet and oral hypoglycaemic agents. He made a good recovery and was discharged home. He failed to attend outpatient follow-up on three occasions and a diabetic liaison sister visited him at home. He was no longer sticking to a diet or taking any medication and he had developed an early diabetic foot ulcer. The diabetic liaison sister, with the district nurse, was able to cure the foot ulcer and regain good diabetic control without recourse to a further hospital admission. Mr Acharya had been under the impression that he suffered from 'very mild diabetes' only and had not seen the need to return to hospital, and he was unaware of the potentially severe complications of diabetes.

Comment

It is very difficult to take a history from a patient who has poor understanding of English. Mr Acharya's pain appeared to have none of the usual characteristics of cardiac pain but he was subsequently shown to have had a definite heart attack. This may have prevented him from receiving specific treatment for a heart attack at an early stage. However, he made an excellent recovery. Again because of language problems he was not educated about his diabetes – the importance of good control and the prevention of complications. Fortunately, follow-up by an enthusiastic liaison nurse remedied this and no serious harm was done.

Fig. 11.1 Checklist for doctors

```
History :
                Use correct full name.
                Use a qualified interpreter if necessary.
                Country of origin: how long in the UK?
                Religion
                Language – main and second language.
                Diet
                Medication
                   – prescribed
                   – herbal remedies, etc.
                International travel

Examination:
                Need to preserve modesty
                Use of chaperone
                Respect for traditional dress
                Need for reassurance

Explanations :  (use an interpreter if necessary)

                Medical procedures
                Medication – short term / long term
                Implications of illness and likely recovery
                Need for blood tests, x-rays etc.
                Role of various therapists
                Aims of treatment
                Follow up arrangements
                Health education advice
                Multi-lingual leaflets to supplement verbal information
```

Conclusion

Physicians, surgeons and psychiatrists need to be alert to the particular needs of ethnic minority elders in the casualty departments, in outpatients, on the wards and following discharge from hospital. The difficulties faced by these vulnerable groups can be overcome with sympathy and tact and if the doctor appreciates and understands the different religions and backgrounds he is likely to encounter. Sympathetic understanding of cultural background is the key to winning patient confidence. A checklist (Fig. 11.1) is useful to avoid overlooking the potential pitfalls. There is still much more research needed in this important area of medical practice.

References

BAXTER, C. (1988). Ethnic minority carers. The invisible carers. *Health and Race*, 15: pp. 4–8.

BRITISH THORACIC AND TUBERCULOSIS ASSOCIATION (1975). Tuberculosis among immigrants related to length of residence in England and Wales. *British Medical Journal*, 3: pp. 698–9.

BURKE, A. W. (1989). Psychiatric practice and ethnic minorities. In CRUICKSHANK, J. K. and BEEVERS, D. G. (eds.) *Ethnic Factors in Health and Disease*, pp. 178–89. John Wright, London.

CRUICKSHANK, J. K. (1989a). Continuing rarity of ischaemic heart disease in Afro-Caribbeans in the West Indies and the UK and in West Africa. In CRUICKSHANK, J. K. and BEEVERS, D. G. (eds.) *Ethnic Factors in Health and Disease*, pp. 264–6. John Wright, London.

CRUICKSHANK, J. K. (1989b). The natural history of blood pressure in black populations. In CRUICKSHANK, J. K. and BEEVERS, D. G. (eds.) *Ethnic Factors in Health and Disease*, pp. 268–79. John Wright, London.

DAVIDSON, A. G., HILDREY, A. C. C. and FLOYER, M. A. (1983). Health problems of ethnic minorities. *British Medical Journal*, **286**: pp. 1575–6.

DONALDSON, L. J. (1986). Health and social status of elderly Asians: a community survey. *British Medical Journal*, **293**: pp. 1079–82.

EDITORIAL (1976). Metabolic bone disease in Asians. *British Medical Journal*, 2: 442–3.

GEORGE, J. and YOUNG, J. B. (1988). Rehabilitation and elderly ethnic minorities. In SQUIRES, A. (ed.) *Rehabilitation of the Older Patient*, pp. 156–66. Croom Helm, London.

HONEY, T. and MATHER, H. M. (1987). Community diabetic clinics and the diabetes specialist nurse. *Practical Diabetes*, 4: pp. 2–4.

HUGHES, L. O. and CRUICKSHANK, J. K. (1989). Ischaemic heart disease in people of Indian subcontinent origin. In CRUICKSHANK, J. K. and BEEVERS, D. G. (eds.) *Ethnic Factors in Health and Disease*, pp. 257–62. John Wright, London.

HUGHES, L. O., RAVAL, V. and RAFTERY, E. B. (1989). Coronary disease in Asians: an ethnic problem. *British Medical Journal*, **298**: pp. 1340–5.

LAWRENCE, R. E. and LITTLER, W. A. (1985). Acute myocardial infarction in Asians and Whites in Birmingham. *British Medical Journal*, **290**: p. 1472.

NORMAN, A. (1985). *Triple Jeopardy: Growing Old in a Second Homeland*. Centre for Policy on Ageing, London.

NICHOLL, C. G., LEVY, J. C., MOHAN, V., RAO, P. V. and MATHER, H. M. (1986). Asian diabetes in Britain: a clinical profile. *Diabetic Medicine*, **3**: 257–60.

ODUGBESAN, O., ROWE, B., FLETCHER, J., WALFORD, S. and BARNETT, A. H. (1989). Diabetes in the UK West Indian community: the Wolverhampton Survey, **6**, pp. 48–52.

PARKER, G. (1985). *With Due Care and Attention: A Review of Research on Informal Care*. Family Policy Studies Centre, London.

SIMMONS, D., WILLIAMS, D. R. R. and POWELL, M. J. (1989). Prevalence of diabetes in a predominantly Asian community: preliminary findings of the Coventry diabetes study. **298**: pp. 18–21.

STEVENS, K. A. and FLETCHER, R. F. (1989). Communicating with Asian patients. *British Medical Journal*, **299**: pp. 905–6.

WOLVERHAMPTON HEALTH AUTHORITY (1989). Asian Language Prevention of Heart Disease leaflet. Health Education Department. Wolverhampton Health Authority, Wolverhampton.

12

Hospital and community nursing of elderly people from ethnic minority groups

Arlene Trim

The diversity of health care demands in multicultural Britain poses an interesting challenge to the unique function of the nurse. In 1973 the International Council of Nurses devised a code of ethics which suggests that, inherent in nursing is respect for life, dignity and the rights of people. These principles are particularly pertinent to the formulation of nursing care for elderly people since they are often marginalised and stripped of their rights, dignity and respect by well meaning care givers. It is important for nurses to keep these issues in the forefront of their minds as they begin to respond to new health care demands both in hospitals and the community. As with most care provision, it is the understanding and attitudes to the problem, rather than a change in clinical skills, which is relevant.

In line with demographic trends elderly ethnic minority people are becoming the recipients of nursing care, in hospitals and in the community, to an increasing extent. The efficiency and effectiveness of this care will depend largely on nurses' ability to demonstrate an awareness and sensitivity to the fact that, in addition to the fundamental difficulties associated with ageing in Western society, ethnic elders face the dilemma of ageing in a foreign country, where inevitably their needs are denied, overlooked or trivialised.

In cases where their needs are identified, the extent to which positive and productive efforts are made to meet these needs are still marginal. It is hoped that the issues raised and explained in this chapter will encourage nurses to look critically at present practice and begin to develop strategies for providing individualised patient care from a multicultural perspective.

Overwhelming evidence suggests that cultural factors determine the extent to which ethnic minority groups perceive, interpret and respond to illness. These factors also contribute significantly to the individual's experience of being a patient.

A patient-centred approach to nursing care will facilitate participation and enable the nurse to work closely with the patient in order to provide a level of care which reflects the needs of the patient and subsequently aids the rehabilitative process. This approach should also help to alleviate the temptation to devise nursing care plans which are based on inaccurate generalisations and stereotypes with little regard for the patient's needs and preferences. In practice it means looking at the individual as a whole, attaching importance to the mental, physical, social and emotional dimensions. In relation to the care of ethnic minority elders it involves the acknowledgement of their past and present experience and knowledge in relation to culture, migration and family life.

The role of the hospital nurse

Essentially, from the hospital nursing perspective, the rehabilitation process begins the moment the patient is admitted. It is a process which involves helping patients to return to their previous capabilities or assisting them to gain the maximum benefit from their existing capabilities. One of the key methods of achieving this, is to ensure that the patient's physical, social and psychological needs are met. This cannot be achieved by nursing intervention alone, but should involve the patient, his or her family, close friends, health care professionals with the necessary expertise and others. The latter might involve voluntary organisations and interest groups which often play an important part in the rehabilitation process especially following discharge from hospital by providing essential supportive services to patients, their families and carers. Increasingly these groups have made significant contributions to the well being of ethnic minority elderly people by providing social networks, nutritious meals, health promotion activities, advice on state benefits and support for carers. Such groups offer a variety of facilities and are invariably acceptable to ethnic elders and their families. Where appropriate they should participate in the planning of long and short term health care goals. Ultimately, however, the final decision should rest with the patient.

There may be marked variations in individual response and reaction to hospitalisation and its consequences, therefore 'blanket' conclusions cannot be drawn. It has been argued that variations in patient behaviour suggest that there is a need for nurses to know about the illness behaviour of the cultures from which their patients are drawn.

Cultural diversity exists even among those of similar racial grouping. It is particularly important for nurses to be aware of this because it might influence the way some ethnic minority elderly people interact and respond to each other in hospital. Hence, introducing two individuals to each other on the ward, placing them in very close proximity or arranging for them to share the same room on the basis that they will communicate and support each other, might prove disastrous in circumstances where caste, religion and other practices are significant contentious factors. Ignorance or indifference to these situations can produce intolerable emotional discomfort for some patients. Similarly, attention should be paid to patients' preferences in relation to personal hygiene, diet, treatment including wound care, taking medicines, blood transfusions, knowledge of acceptable language, use of a hospital interpreter – to name but a few issues – in order to provide culture sensitive individualised care.

The need for a knowledge base

In order to minimise misunderstanding it is essential that nurses are adequately prepared and equipped to care for ethnic minority elders. This cannot be adequately achieved, without access to a flexible culture specific body of knowledge. This should evolve from careful, accurate documentation and research. The personal resource that nurses from ethnic minorities possess should not be overlooked, and recruitment from this source encouraged. Staff training in transcultural health care should be an ongoing process within the hospital setting. Post registration training involving contact with minority groups should be encouraged, as should comprehensive in-service education.

It should also form part of a cohesive strategy for health care provision for ethnic minority groups as a whole, and be included in all nurse education curricula.

Gaps in the knowledge of staff members should not be seen as a personal deficit; instead they should be used to generate new knowledge. This can be achieved by encouraging individuals to pursue areas of interest or to try new ideas – for example, flexible, culture sensitive assessment procedures can be devised (Baxter, 1988). Subsequently when they have been tried and evaluated they can be implemented in a ward or department. This initiative is only one of many which can develop as a result of a recognition of the need to fulfil a gap in knowledge.

The responsibility for collecting and distilling information should not be left to any one group, however. It should be a collective effort involving all personnel who contribute to the care of ethnic minority elders. Health authorities, hospital trusts and other managerial bodies, have a distinct responsibility to provide appropriate care for the people they serve. This can only be achieved if more effort is made to respond to issues relating to the health of ethnic minority elders. Implementation of the Association of Health Authorities Working Party recommendations would be a positive step.

Relevant, up to date information should be available to staff, accompanied by appropriate in-service education and guidance. Evidence of a shift of focus from mortality statistics, which provide useful but limited information to those directly involved in providing nursing care for ethnic minority elders, should be seen. In addition, more emphasis should be placed on the interpretation and analysis of morbidity statistics. For instance, evidence suggests that diabetes and hypertension are often the major causes of ill health and death among Afro-Caribbeans. Morbidity statistics will highlight the incidence and rate of onset of resulting degenerative disabilities such as poor eyesight, reduced circulation and strokes. Such information can be extremely useful because it may form the basis on which screening programmes and follow-up care facilities are based.

Issues relating to quality of life, including environmental and other influencing factors, ought to be addressed in more detail. Invariably, these issues have a direct bearing on the health of the individual. Clear statements relating to long and short term goals for health promotion and screening should be made where appropriate. Nurses should be invited to participate, and contribute to the planning and implementation of strategies necessary to achieve these goals. Recognition and utilisation of the knowledge and expertise of legitimate representatives of ethnic minority elderly people could go a long way towards improving standards and providing patient centred care in hospital. In areas where there are very few ethnic minority elderly residents, nurses should be given the opportunity to develop an awareness of programmes and initiatives which are implemented in areas where the group form a substantial part of the total population. Undoubtedly, there is a need for nurses to feel confident and comfortable to critically analyse and explore sensitive issues relating to culture, race, prejudice, religion and sexuality. Opportunities for the exploration of personal feelings in an atmosphere of trust, ought to give nurses an insight into their own attitudes and values in relation to the areas mentioned above. It is difficult to eliminate poor practice if professionals inadvertently create, nurture and maintain it.

Innovations in nursing care for ethnic minority groups are beginning to emerge.

Baxter (1988) suggests that the use of a checklist which covers sensitive areas relating to foods, religion, diet, hygiene, death and bereavement can provide guidance for nurses and assist in the development of a systematic approach to information gathering. The efficacy and legitimacy of these practices can only be substantiated by frequent evaluation and improvement. There is also a call for the development of transcultural nursing research which can be used to inform practice.

An example of the need to gain information around the issue of hygiene can be demonstrated by the following religious preferences.

- Muslims prefer to wash in free flowing water rather than in a bath. They need water in toilets and toilet paper is not considered adequate. The left hand is traditionally used to wash the private parts and the right hand is used for eating. When handing something to a Muslim it is courteous to use the right hand. This custom is shared with other people from the Indian subcontinent.
- Every Muslim must wash thoroughly before praying. This ritual wash follows a set routine and running water is required.
- After menstruation, Muslim women are required to wash their whole bodies.
- Hindus will need water for washing in the toilet. Hindu patients much prefer to wash in free flowing water rather than sitting in a bath. A shower is often preferable.
- Sikhs prefer to wash in free flowing water and require water for washing in the toilet. Sitting in a bath is not considered an adequate means of cleansing the body. A shower is preferable.

The use of skills

Efforts to provide patient-centred care to ethnic minority elders will be severely undermined if, as nurses, we fail to see the need to link other important skills to the process. For example, communication skills involving open and closed questions can assist in an assessment procedure. The use of a skilful sensitive questioning technique can enable the nurse to gain some insight into the patient's expectations and anxieties. These skills also facilitate dialogue between the patient, relatives and the nurse.

Listening is another valuable skill which can be used to convey to patients and their relatives or carers that they are heard and that what they have said is respected. Genuine, appropriate verbal and non-verbal responses can convey a number of positive messages. Competencies such as clear diction, accuracy and attention to detail especially in relation to the explanations and implementation of nursing procedures are essential to the maintenance of acceptable standards of care in hospital.

Closely linked to the skills and competencies mentioned above is the ability to work closely and effectively with interpreters. In cases where there are difficulties with verbal communication, discreet use of the services of known interpreters can be invaluable. Details of their location should be available to all nursing staff. A reduction in the incidence of misunderstanding and fear can be sustained, if procedures are explained to patients in a language which both they and their interpreters can understand.

Strategies for feedback, to ensure that the correct messages are being transmitted, have to be developed and evaluated in order to provide scope for modification and change in keeping with patients' needs.

The role of the extended family

Observation of the interaction between elderly patients and their family can give the nurse some indication of the level of stress and anxiety they may be experiencing. Accurate assessment of the behaviour and interaction of family members cannot be achieved from a brief interaction with them. For example, there is often a temptation to draw conclusions on admission. It is important to realise that often this is the most stressful period for patients themselves and for their families. Illness and subsequent hospitalisation of a relative can alter the family dynamics. On admission patients may display a change of behaviour precipitated by discomfort, confusion and fear. This may have a direct effect on their response and interaction with family members. This apparent change of behaviour, if met with a lack of understanding, can give rise to hostility and impatience.

The nurse's assessment of family dynamics can be assisted by flexible observation, reinforced by continued verbal interactions with patients and their relatives who must be given the opportunity to acknowledge and explore their own feelings. The nurse might not be in a position to facilitate this exploration however. An accurate assessment of the situation should highlight areas of need and, if necessary, an appropriate referral can be made to a counsellor or relevant supportive organisation. Link workers who are trained to deal with these situations can be introduced to the family who should then be given the opportunity to decide whether the input of a supportive network will be relevant to their needs; but they should not feel pressured to accept the service.

The co-operation of family members is essential to the smooth implementation of the rehabilitation process (Boroch, 1976). This can only be achieved if they are made to feel part of the treatment process, without compromising the individuality, dignity and confidentiality of the patient. The family has a part to play in promoting positive health outcomes for the ill person. Positive responses from them can help their relative to develop confidence in the professionals who are responsible for his or her care in hospital. Often, however, the needs and expectations of the family are unintentionally overlooked or ignored. This is especially true in cases where an imbalance between what the family is capable of offering in terms of economic, physical, emotional and psychological support to their relative and the expectations of the health and social services personnel occurs. This imbalance may be compounded by the patient's own expectations of relatives, which is often based on past experience of elderly people in their country of origin.

In England, there is no uniformity among ethnic minority elderly people with regard to their status and roles in second or even third generation family units. Clark *et al.* (1984) found that a significant number of elderly Asians lived with their children and grandchildren. Donaldson and Odell (1984) found that living with the extended family did have some disadvantages. Privacy was limited, and in some cases social and emotional needs were not fully met. Often this was not due to deliberate negligence by the family. On the contrary, the situation was often created by circumstances beyond their control – such as social, economic and environmental factors. These determine the extent to which the extended family can provide facilities which could enable their elderly relatives to enjoy optimum, social, physical, emotional and psychological well being. Barker (1984) found that a significant number of elderly people from ethnic minority groups choose to live alone, but those who had children expressed the need to see them frequently. These findings show that, although the elderly valued their privacy and independence, they derived great pleasure from contact with their children.

Although changes in the availability of employment and housing have generated increased mobility among second and third generation ethnic minority groups, regular contact with elderly relatives is maintained (in most cases) by visits and telephone contacts. Despite the fact that the input may be limited by circumstances, a significant number of elderly people from ethnic minority groups still receive a substantial amount of help and support from their children and extended family. More research is needed in this area to determine how much of the responsibility for the care of elderly relatives rests on the shoulders of the extended family. Evidence suggests that an increasing number of elderly people are living alone and have very little contact with relatives. Instead they rely heavily on friends, neighbours and statutory services for help and support. A high percentage of the group is comprised of women who are widowed, single or separated and these may be drawn from a range of ethnic backgrounds including Polish, German, Asian, Irish and Afro-Caribbean, to name but a few. Some are disadvantaged by failure to utilise fully the statutory services available to all elderly people in this country. This may be due to the fact that the services are not accessible to them, they are unaware of their rights or, it may be that what is provided fails to meet their needs. This is particularly true of Asian and Afro-Caribbean elderly (Bhalla and Blakemore, 1981; Donaldson, 1986). Contrary to popular belief, ethnic minority elders are quite willing to use appropriate supportive services. 90 per cent of the elderly Asians in a sample were willing to attend social clubs which provided the opportunity to meet others of like backgrounds and interests. In this group men tended to go out more frequently than women. These issues only serve to reinforce the importance of individual assessments which should assist in determining patients' needs on a personal level.

It would be futile for nurses to contribute to a rehabilitative programme for ethnic minority elderly patients based on the assumption that they are the recipients of adequate and consistent family support. In cases where families are willing to take an active part in the rehabilitative programme of their elderly relatives, they should be given the opportunity to discuss their own needs and anxieties. Sensitive areas relating to accommodation and finance may be discussed in a non-threatening, non-intrusive manner. Often the patient remains the focus of attention and family members are ignored. They may reinforce the situation by encouraging carers to concentrate on their ill relative simply by indicating that his or her welfare is the main priority. This attitude can mask a range of concerns, for instance, there may be anxieties about taking an elderly relative home following a stroke, because the family do not know how to cater for his or her daily needs. They may not be familiar with the supportive services in the community, or provision of equipment and modification of existing accommodation at no cost to them. Care should be taken, therefore, to ensure that relevant information is given and continuing support for the family is maintained. At the same time they should be able to acknowledge and come to terms with the fact that they might not be in a position to provide the appropriate care and facilities for the elderly relative because of the nature of his or her disability.

Acknowledging primary carers

In 1985 the writer conducted a small pilot study to identify the health needs of elderly Afro-Caribbean in a London Borough. One third of the respondents were disabled by strokes, one had severe rheumatoid arthritis accompanied by restricted movement. In all of the cases, the main carer was an elderly husband or wife. In cases where district nurses and other statutory carers were involved, partners were responsible for a major proportion of the care. These findings are in keeping with the national trends which highlight the needs of carers throughout the United Kingdom. Elderly partners were providing the main proportion of care for the frail elderly. They also found that the distribution of responsibility was equal between male and female carers. In most cases care is perceived as a labour of love but, increasingly, the difficulties experienced by primary carers are highlighted. These include a high level of physical, emotional, and economic stress. Health profession-als are encouraged to demonstrate an awareness of difficulties that carers experience. Every effort should be made to ensure that carers are given the advice and support they need. Ethnic minority primary carers may be disadvantaged in a number of ways apart from those mentioned. They may be unaware of the services which are available in hospital and the community to assist them in carrying out their roles effectively. They should be aware of the facilities available from some voluntary and statutory agencies. Information about monetary benefits, mechanical aids, community nursing input, night sitting services, dial-a-ride, and support groups for carers should be offered in ways which encourages them to feel confident enough to take up the services when appropriate.

Information and support to primary carers should be an essential part of the role of the hospital nurse. In times of crisis or intense activity it is easy for health personnel to focus their attention and liaise with the younger perhaps more articulate family members. This may be appropriate in some family circumstances with elderly relatives, especially in cases where there is a limited knowledge of English or the bureaucratic system, but this approach cannot be applied in all situations. Elderly carers who have no children or extended families should be involved in setting the nursing care goals which are aimed at facilitating the rehabilitative process. All activities should be explained carefully, anxieties should be aired and liaison with professional colleagues in the community should be made in order to facilitate continuity of care.

Another important issue involves choice in relation to accommodation. Many ethnic minority elderly people prefer to live at home with their partners rather than share with their children or extended family. Sheltered accommodation is another choice which can be taken up. Hitherto some such arrangements have been unsuitable due to lack of sensitivity and understanding by indigenous white residents and service providers.

Increasingly housing associations which are located in areas where there are large numbers of ethnic minority elderly residents are providing warden controlled and other purpose built accommodation for them. This is illustrated by work initiated by Birmingham Friendship Housing Association, Asians Sheltered Residential Accommodation (ASRA), and the Carib Housing Association. These are just a few of the known associations which are currently providing accommodation for elderly Asians and Afro-Caribbean, similar organisations are providing services for other ethnic groups. Demand is high especially since the amenities are built to a high standard and elderly residents have the added advantage of mutual support from peers with similar backgrounds and experiences.

Using a theoretical framework

Within recent years nurses have been using a number of theoretical frameworks to help them in the planning and practice of care. This is due to increased responsibility to demonstrate a high standard of practice which is closely linked to quality and accountability. Such issues have assumed a new meaning since greater emphasis is placed on the importance of consumer needs and demands.

A number of nursing models have been develped and utilised to encompass the above concepts – Orem's self-care model, the Roy adaptation model, Neuman's health care systems model and Roy's adaptation model based on the activities of daily living are just a few. It is important to acknowledge their importance because, as McFarlane (1986) points out, conceptual models link theory to practice and are thus extremely useful to nursing practice. They also give rise to new theories and concepts. As the emphasis on individualised care increases nurses will be expected to draw on a sound theoretical foundation from which to formulate their practice. This is particularly pertinent when they contribute functional assessment criteria for use in the rehabilitation of ethnic minority elders. The model based on the activities of daily living has been developed and reviewed by Roper, Logan and Tierney (1981). The writer believes that the content of this model can be utilised and adapted to form a useful assessment tool from which to identify needs and problems during the rehabilitation period. It allows the team to set long and short term achievable goals based on the activities of daily living which are observable, measurable phenomena that patients and their carers can understand and relate to. The nurse is then able to plan, implement and review care in a clear systematic way.

Roper *et al.* (1981) point out that these activities of daily living are complex and closely related, but they can be considered in the variety of circumstances in relation to the needs of the patient, for instance, maintaining a safe environment. Ethnic minority patients with strokes, going through the first phase of the rehabilitative process in hospital, may be very fearful of trying to stand with an aid. Loss of feeling in one or two limbs may provoke a profound sense of despair exaggerated by fear of not being able to cope with a walking aid and support from the nurse. Here, an awareness of the patient's own interpretation of his or her illness would help. For example, patients are less likely to co-operate if they feel their illness to be a punishment from God which they should accept. The nurse can accept such a belief, while helping the patient to see that loss of function in one or two limbs does not mean that he or she cannot regain some degree of independence. When the model provides a framework on which to base nursing practice, the process of nursing will provide a systematic approach to care that will help to highlight and evaluate the nursing input.

Looking again at the example based on the patient's interpretation of illness, such an attitude will invariably influence motivation. Nurses who are able to facilitate an exploration of the patient's feelings are more likely to be able to assess his or her level of motivation and be able to plan a programme of care which takes this issue into account. As the patient becomes more or less confident, the care plan can be adapted and re-evaluated. The nurse can help the patient to recognise and value his or her own achievements. As the patient's confidence grows, he or she begins to regain self-confidence and confidence in the environment. Increasing the individual's responsibility for his or her own safety should be encouraged and measured in terms of the appropriate use of equipment, adherence to guidelines relating to getting in and out of bed and general mobilisation.

There are no fixed rules with regard to the choice and utilisation of nursing models, although it is well known and documented that some can be adapted to specific situations better than others. It is essential that the key elements of any model are examined carefully to ensure that it is suitable for use with a particular patient. In some cases elements from two nursing models can be used to assist in the development of a comprehensive care plan which recognises the patient's needs, not only in terms of physical activities but emotional and environmental issues.

Communication is another very important activity of living which can be explored. It should not be assessed merely on the ability of the patient to understand English but, rather, should involve ascertaining whether the patient is literate and can read and write in their own language. It should also involve understanding and responding to the verbal and non-verbal cues of English speaking ethnic minority elderly people. This approach should form the basis for partnership between the patient and the nurse, and should also assist in the evaluation process.

Patients who are able to communicate effectively are more likely to express their preferences with regard to their health care goals.

The role of the health visitor

Over the years health visitors have been actively involved in the health care of elderly people in the community. Some health authorities employ specialist health visitors whose sole remit is to visit the elderly. Others employ registered general nurses as geriatric visitors. Many health visitors welcome this initiative because they acknowledge that limited resources and increasing demands for health care inhibit their ability to provide the level of care they consider worthwhile and acceptable for elderly people in the community. Others recognise ageing as a natural part of life's continuum and are actively involved in the care of the elderly. They are supported by their employing authority and members of the health care team. Health visitors have been able to demonstrate that caring for the elderly can be an important aspect of health visiting practice, providing ample scope for health promotion. More research would have to be undertaken to assess the value of health visitor involvement in the rehabilitation of the elderly. Where geriatricians acknowledge the value of health visiting input with the elderly after their discharge from hospital, appropriate referrals result in more health visitor involvement with the severely disabled.

Health visitor involvement with ethnic minority elderly

There is very little research available which looks specifically at health visitor input with ethnic minority elderly. This may be due to lack of awareness or to deficits in the referral system between hospital and the community and between general practitioners and the community nursing service (Baxter *et al.*, 1988). This situation should improve as health visitors become more involved in teamwork and other professionals become more aware of their role. Health visitors are beginning to become involved in health education and surveillance activities. Health promotion among the middle aged and younger elderly should bring health visitors in closer contact with ethnic minority elder people since those who arrived in England in the 1950s and 1960s will be approaching old age at this time. There is tremendous scope for the development of further research into the health needs of ethnic minority elderly people. The information which is available today can be used as a starting point from which health visitors and district nurses can identify areas where their expertise can be utilised effectively for the benefit of ethnic minority elderly consumers. Evidence suggests that there is a high incidence of morbidity from arthritis, strokes, raised blood pressure and heart disease, hence they are more likely to be the recipients of comprehensive rehabilitative programmes. Pyke Lees and Gardiner (1974) point out that the multiplicity of needs which some ethnic minority elders face often lead to the simultaneous involvement of a number of agencies. In such cases, effective teamwork is important and necessary to ensure that contributions from some disciplines do not become submerged or ignored. It is important to ensure that accurate assessments are carried out and appropriate referrals made which reflect an understanding of the level of input that health visitors can make to the rehabilitative process. A team approach is essential, no one discipline is capable of dealing with the 'whole' individual. For this approach to be effective there should be regular communication and sharing of ideas. In cases where information has to be shared the client and carers should be informed; this helps to ensure that there is some uniformity in the care plan and that clients and their carers are not receiving conflicting advice. Long and short term goals should be set and each discipline should monitor its own input. As the goals are achieved systematic withdrawal of professional input will ensure that the client is given the opportunity to lead as normal a life as possible. Health visitors may have a long term involvement with the client and his or her carers, giving anticipatory advice and support on a range of health related issues. They can utilise their interpersonal skills, knowledge of secondary and tertiary care, awareness of resources in the community and their ability to liaise with other agencies, to assist in the co-ordination of resources which will ultimately benefit the client.

Apart from health professionals and other agencies, health visitors have to develop other strategies for reaching ethnic minority elderly people in the community. The identification of minority groups is a sensitive issue and has already been discussed; sensitivity must be employed.

Age/sex registers can be very useful if they have some means of identifying ethnic minority elders. Ethnicity and country of origin should be clearly stated. The use of 'community profiles' which clearly identify the ethnic groups, their age, sex, family structure, housing status, their health needs supported by mortality and morbidity statistics could be developed. The number of carers can also be identified – their age, sex and the type of responsibility should be stated, recreational and voluntary organisations relevant to the group should also be noted. These are just a few of the areas which can be highlighted in the community profile, which can be developed with the help of the latest population census. OPCS statistical data, health authority reports and long term strategies for care in the community information from local churches and voluntary organisations can assist the health visitor to identify ethnic minority elderly people in the community.

Where appropriate, direct contact with potential clients can be organised. Strategies for the encouragement of self referral can also be developed by providing information about the health care services in the community, in local libraries, luncheon clubs and other organisations attended by ethnic minority elders.

There is no doubt that health visitors can make a significant and important contribution to the rehabilitation of ethnic minority elders in the community. This can be achieved by giving support and information to carers. Health teaching sessions can be organised and carried out in suitable premises to groups of individuals. These sessions can be geared to help elderly people to take responsibility for their own health care and to seek help if their present condition deteriorates or as soon as they recognise any deviation from the norm. They can be encouraged to participate in screening programmes geared to detect the early onset of debilitative conditions.

In cases where individuals are disabled there is a lot of scope in health visiting practice for helping clients to adjust to their disability. To achieve these initiatives professional collaboration is essential, therefore, the health visitor would need to liaise with general practitioners, physiotherapists, occupational therapists, district nurses, social workers, voluntary workers and others to devise workable health care goals with the client. This is an ongoing process which has to be examined in the light of current demographic and political trends.

The role of the district nurse

Rehabilitation of patients in the community will take on a greater dimension, more importance will be attached to this aspect of care because of current changes in health care provision. Baly (1981) acknowledges that district nurses make a significant and important contribution to patient rehabilitation. The process is complex for a number of reasons, the most important being the need to elicit the full co-operation of patients and their families. District nurses are invariably confronted by the formidable task of helping to motivate people who often have multiple medical and social problems. They are also expected to liaise with other professionals.

There is a high incidence of morbidity among ethnic minority elders. A substantial number of those who came to join their families, and others who arrived in England in the 1970s as refugees, are now older and potentially in need of statutory care. The district nurse is in a position to become actively involved in assessing, planning, implementing and evaluating care for this group. To ensure that appropriate provision and support services are available, the district nurse must liaise with other care professionals, mainly general practitioners, physiotherapists, occupational therapists, chiropodists, health visitors, social workers and others. Again the importance of the team approach, economic and effective use of individual expertise cannot be over emphasised. Priorities among team members may change because of shifts of responsibility which may be triggered by the implementation of new ways of working. Pertinent examples include the GP contracts and the introduction of the neighbourhood nursing concept.

District nurses and other health care professionals will not be able to provide ethnic minority elderly clients with the care they deserve if they are unaware of their existence. Badger and colleagues (1988) emphasise the fact that district nurses are often unaware of the health needs of ethnic minority elders in the community who are coping with multiple disabilities and could benefit from district nursing input. The researchers suggest that the reasons for this situation may be linked to the fact that assumptions are made – by general practitioners, district nurses and others – that ethnic minority communities are self-sufficient in relation to the provision of care for the elderly. As a result of such assumptions, very few referrals are made and potential patients continue to suffer.

Undoubtedly there is a need for district nurses to be proactive and devise strategies for identifying patients in need of their expertise in the community.

Case study: Mrs Douglas

Mrs Douglas is a 60 year old Afro-Caribbean woman who came to England in 1963 to work in what she described as 'the rag trade'. After ten years she married a Afro-Caribbean from her own country; they had two children both of whom are now married and living in the United States.

Mrs Douglas lives in a warm, well-maintained first floor flat with two bedrooms and central heating, which is owned by a local housing association. She has lived alone since her husband died two years ago, but has regular contact with her children in America and other relatives in Jamaica by letter and telephone. She has one friend aged 65, who attends the same local church and visits her regularly. Mrs Douglas has planned to return to Jamaica for a holiday in three months time; she has not been home for 20 years so she is looking forward to the holiday.

Mrs Douglas was referred to the district nurse following discharge from hospital after three weeks as an in patient and the diagnosis of insulin-dependent diabetes. She was very shocked by the diagnosis. While she was hospitalised every effort was made to teach her to administer her insulin injections. Depression, disbelief at the sudden change in her health status, together with fear of the unknown, has resulted in her inability to administer her own insulin.

Comment

The district nurse will be expected to recognise the patient's perception of herself and her illness. It would be useful to devise some achievable goals with the patient. Care should be taken to ensure that her emotional, physical and social needs are met. The use of a nursing model (for example, an assessment of Mrs Douglas within the framework of the Activities of Living) would help the nurse to concentrate on key areas relating to the patient, her health and environment including her supportive network. The district nurse would be expected to take a detailed history before assessing specific areas. For example, 'maintaining a safe environment' would involve looking at what the patient cannot do for herself and exploring the underlying fears and anxieties before focusing on the fact that she is unable to administer the insulin herself. Achievable goals could include a gradual introduction to preparation for giving the insulin as well as the removal and safe disposal of syringes and other equipment. Evaluation of the patient's response and execution of these tasks should be carried out. Then a sensitive introduction to self-administration of insulin can be started. Care must be taken to ensure that the dosage is understood and the links with diet – especially in relation to carbohydrate – must be discussed in detail. Eating and drinking can be assessed separately to facilitate the introduction of an exchange system which could include consideration of culture-specific dietary habits. An assessment of working and leisure activities would give Mrs Douglas an opportunity to discuss any anxieties concerning her forthcoming holiday, for example she may be apprehensive about travelling and wonder how that would affect her condition. A full exploration of these anxieties would help the patient to regain her confidence and independence.

Conclusion

Nursing care of ethnic minority elderly people, whether in hospital or in the community, is a worthwhile undertaking which will continue to need careful planning and effective collaboration to move forward with a changing population. Activities should be planned on the basis of a sound understanding and knowledge of the needs of the community served.

References

BARKER, J. (1984). Black and Asian old people in Britain. First report of a research study: Age concern research unit.

BADGER, F. *et al.* (1988). Put race on the agenda (failure of district nursing services to meet the needs of elderly Black people). *Health Service Journal*, **98**: Dec. pp. 1426–7.

BALY, M. (ed.) (1981). *A New Approach to District Nursing*, pp. 144–6. Heinemann Medical Books, London.

BAXTER *et al.* (1988). Racial inequalities in health, a challenge to the British National Health Service. *International Journal of Health Service*, **18** (4): pp. 563–71.

BHALLA, A. and BLAKEMORE, K. (1981). Elders of the minority ethnic groups.

CLARKE, M., CLARKE, S. *et al.* (1984). The elderly at home, health and social status. *Health Trends*, **16**: pp. 3–7.

DONALDSON, L. J. (1986). Health and social status of elderly Asians: a Community Survey. *British Medical Journal*, **293**: pp. 1079–82.

DONALDSON, L. J. and ODELL, A. (1984). Aspects of the health and social needs of elderly Asians in Leicester: a Community Survey. Department of Community Medicine, Leicester.

MCFARLANE J. (1976). The role of research and the development of nursing theory. *Journal of Advanced Nursing*, 1: pp. 443–51.

PYKE LEES, C. and GARDINER, S. (1974). Elderly ethnic minorities. Age Concern, UK.

ROPER, N., LOGAN, W. and TIERNEY, A. (1981). *Learning to Use the Process of Nursing*. Churchill Livingstone.

ROPER *et al*. (1981). The Roper Logan Tierney model. *Senior Nurse*, 3 (1): pp. 20–27. ROTHWELL, T. (1980). General practice ethnicity and service delivery, in *Social Science and Medicine*, 19 (2): pp. 123–30.

13

Physiotherapy with ethnic minority elders

Margaret Heatley and Amanda Squires

The title of this chapter is purposely chosen as physiotherapy has minimal effect without the co-operation of the patient; and with elderly people, for whom mobility and function are frequently the goals, co-operation is essential. To gain this co-operation the perception and goals of the physiotherapist, patient and carer must remain in unison. This chapter aims to outline the development of physiotherapy and current practice, to explore its relevance to ethnic minority elders, and to identify areas where perceptions may differ, and to suggest solutions.

Sociological issues affecting physiotherapy with ethnic minority elders

The necessity to understand the issues relating to the special needs of the ethnic minority population are an increasing obligation of the physiotherapy profession, particularly in the inner city health authorities.

Physiotherapy is the identification and assessment of musculoskeletal and neuromuscular disorders of function including pain, and those of psychosomatic origin, as well as the response to and prevention of those problems by natural methods based essentially on movement and manual therapy (Williams, 1986). Physiotherapy also has a significant part to play in health promotion.

Physiotherapy has its origins in massage, Swedish remedial exercise, physical education, light and electrotherapy (Parry, 1990). The emphasis at the beginning was on improvement in acute conditions to enable the person to return to a chosen occupation. The profession has probably incorporated more traditional medicine – such as massage, hydrotherapy and acupuncture – than any other in the National Health Service. The desire to improve practice based on scientific evaluation has brought advancement of technology and an increased clinical/scientific approach to treatment planning.

Physiotherapy in rehabilitation of the elderly developed after the Second World War when the depravities of the 'workhouse' had been revealed by evacuation. At this time, demobilised PT instructors who had trained as physiotherapists for the war effort were available to assist rehabilitation (Squires, 1986). The development of the National Health Service in 1947 meant that access to free health care was available to all who had the time to wait, not just the wealthy, insured or employed. Elderly people had possibly the most to gain from the creation of the NHS.

With this background, and the need to keep as many elderly people in their chosen environment as possible, the emphasis was on rehabilitation, and it is only in relatively recent years that the physiotherapy contribution to chronic and terminal illness in all age groups has been recognised. The work of agencies such as Age Concern has done much to break down ageist attitudes. This has encouraged the young elderly to have higher expectations, thereby helping to promote the use of physiotherapy. In many cases, however, the old elderly reflect the views of an earlier era.

Increased media coverage has increased the profile of what is available to elderly people, this includes adventurous holidays such as SAGA, dedicated magazines such as *Choice* and exercise programmes such as EXTEND.

Physiotherapy has a tradition of respect from the public. Unfortunately the 'white coat' image has created an expectation of passive cure. The reality of the physiotherapy task is to motivate the person to participate in his or her own recovery – which can give the reputation of effort and discomfort.

The British-born elderly who have lived alongside the development of the profession have, therefore, an image of physiotherapy for acute conditions in the young and middle aged. The tradition of independence and fear of the workhouse which was the only accommodation for the indigent, isolated old, has developed in them a spirit of independence with which the physiotherapist can work to maintain and improve mobility and enable life to be lived in the person's chosen environment.

Physiotherapy in all countries moves with the stage of economic development, health care system, social attitudes and the life expectancy of its population. Developing countries will probably focus more on the basic needs of survival highlighted by nutritional and immunisation programmes, whilst more developed countries may emphasise high technology survival. Health care provision varies between national public, insurance based or mixed systems of financing. There may be quite different systems for urban and rural areas in geographically large countries with widely spread population and transport difficulties. Social attitudes may direct care to the curable and/or to those with chronic problems. Life expectancy will determine whether an elderly population exists in any significant number, and population trends will indicate the availability of carers.

It should be remembered that in developing countries not only is life expectancy lower, but biological ageing is faster and morbidity such as malnutrition and infection leading to death are not influenced by physiotherapy. This means both that the consequences of ageing occur earlier (such as senile dementia in 50 year olds), and that morbidity from a Westernised lifestyle will more likely be the consequence of cerebrovascular and cardiovascular disease, which are rehabilitable, and with which first generation ethnic minority elders have little acquaintance.

Ageist policies may respect, or just accept, this section of the population. Physiotherapy, therefore, will differ in each country studied and an understanding of all these factors will be necessary to appreciate the attitudes and expectations of patients from minority cultures.

Social skills between client and therapist also require consideration. A welfare system necessitates basic courtesy and a compliant patient; surroundings are of little consequence as there is little choice – and the neighbouring hospital is probably little different. An insurance-based system puts the client in charge; courtesy is paramount to gain future custom and surroundings are congenial. Therefore patients accustomed to choice will find the current National Health Service system different from their experience. The future may well be different again.

The process of physiotherapy

Expectation of the components of physiotherapy may also differ. Undressing for a full examination by someone who is not a doctor; active involvement in treatment rather than passive receiving; the scarcity of massage but the availability of acupuncture may be as welcome a surprise to some, as it is frightening to others. Electrotherapy may be expected or feared. In some cultures nearly all physiotherapy treatment programmes have an electrical component and this will be expected – a programme without it will be regarded as inferior.

The interest of the family in the various procedures may also vary. Some Asian relatives may be used to spending all day in the hospital helping with the patient as necessary, and providing food. The attendance of up to three generations around the bed is expected, with the presence of children essential. In Britain since the Second World War the family has been protected more and more from the realities of illness and death. This is not necessarily so elsewhere and presence at a procedure or at death may be expected by both patient and relatives. Being faced with 'Visiting Times 2–4 pm, only two visitors to a bed and no children' on some British wards can be a shock to visitor and patient alike. The relaxation of these rules and the encouragement of visitors, at least to the physiotherapy department, where space may be more available, can be an excellent public relations exercise from which the profession and patient can only benefit.

A similar enthusiasm for visiting may occur when the patient attends the outpatient department or day hospitals. Facilities should be available and the relevant family members included in the treatment programme wherever possible.

The social nature of nationalities also varies. The traditional reserve of the indigenous British may mean that patients in adjacent beds for weeks may only acknowledge each other daily by surnames. Encouraging those who wish to converse with others will also go some way to breaking down barriers and encouraging mutual exchange of knowledge. This may be spontaneous, but sensitive introductions can be made by staff and communication allowed to develop. Some nationalities are more outgoing and find this reserve offensive. Physical touch is expected in some cultures, in others it is open to misrepresentation. Physiotherapists, by the nature of their work, are 'touchers' and need to be alert to how this action is being received. Patients from some cultures are also 'touchers' and may regard an embrace at the end of a treatment as quite normal – to the surprise of the therapist.

The development of communities of minority ethnic groups is a natural phenomenon. People in adversity help each other, and in the face of over-whelming difficulties of knowledge, access, communication, etc., self-help groups develop. These may have as their stimulus age, religion, disease, or cultural interests and may be eligible to access local funding. Where these have evolved for the support of ethnic minority elderly, they provide a focus which physiotherapists should use to enable health promotion, accident prevention advice, and general information on mobility and function to enable independence to be pursued if desired. They can also be used to prevent misguided enthusiasm from the misinformed.

Physiotherapy may have quite a different status in the eyes of the public, being seen at one extreme as 'labour' and therefore of low status, and on the other hand as only undertaken by those medically qualified – as in Russia where an additional course has to be undertaken after graduation in medicine. Access to the service may also vary. In countries where State provision is scare, a flourishing private market may exist and, indeed, may be virtually the only source of physiotherapy. Does the patient in Britain realise that NHS treatment is being provided free? In some cultures, such as the Chinese community, private medicine is seen to be superior and this attitude may have travelled with the patient. The autonomy of the profession also varies. In the United Kingdom the physiotherapist diagnoses the clinical problem and plans, carries out or directs appropriate intervention. In some countries prescriptive treatment is still practised, particularly where doctor-physiotherapists use lesser or unqualified staff to carry out the activity. This approach may confuse any patient used to another system.

The model of physiotherapy may also vary. The British system of preventing admission, or aiming at discharge with transport provided for outpatient appointments, may be contrasted with extensive countries with large rural populations where admission is the requirement for access to a total rehabilitation programme due to the difficulties of transport for outpatient appointments. It is crucial for the family to be taught to continue the programme.

Even in extensive countries, living near access to outpatient facilities may enable attendance but transport may have to be paid for by the patient, as in India. Does the patient understand that failure to admit, or plans for discharge, do not necessarily mean that access to physiotherapy is denied? Could failure of outpatient attendance be linked to this – had anyone thought of explaining?

Consideration should also be given to the increasing generation gap found between ethnic minority elders and their offspring. The demands of the older person for traditional support within the family unit may not be matched by the result of the influence of western culture on the younger family members.

The non-indigenous elderly therefore have various expectations of physiotherapy in addition to their own health beliefs. Has physiotherapy been heard of? Is its function clear? Is the status of the physiotherapist seen as a doctor or auxiliary? Will discharge occur only when the person is fully rehabilitated? Will the family – who may not be available – be expected to carry on? Will outpatient attendance mean paying for transport? Is the walking aid/appliance/wheelchair to be paid for? Does rehabilitation mean that return to work is expected? Is the treatment private and does it need to be paid for? Why should I bother anyway when my family is there and has been brought up to look after me?

In many cases, therefore, first generation 'old elderly' from ethnic minorities are in a different era although the degree of this will vary. Some may have been living in Britain for 50 years. Others may have been catapulted into current practices having arrived recently as dependants of children already settled. Their expectations of life and of physiotherapy may be compared with the early 1950s in Britain, but their families' expectations are of the 1990s as are those of members of the team.

Physiotherapists who work with patients from cultures different from their own are faced with the dilemma of meeting the demands of the service, the team, the client and their own learned expectations. Job satisfaction can only be gained when expectations of all concerned are aired openly. The differing expectations of different members of the team also need consideration. Some members may have expectations based on other experiences, other cultures, or other systems. The value of physiotherapy with this group may be misinterpreted and, for a successful outcome, perceptions and expectations must be clarified. All must be aired and shared.

If the cultural norms of families (and therefore their children as potential student members of the health care professions) do not appreciate rehabilitation but focus on family care alone; if careers teachers lack appreciation of physiotherapy, student recruitment may be compromised and the profession will continue to have a relatively small ethnic membership. The physiotherapy department frequently has the strength of cultural diversity in its helper staff group, who being recruited locally can reflect the mix of the population, their culture and perhaps their language.

It is seen that there are many issues that can be misinterpreted, and as many reasons for discouraging co-operation in the hope that physiotherapy will cease and the problems it could raise can be ignored.

Clinical issues for physiotherapists with ethnic minority elders

Physiotherapists are trained to see the whole patient in his or her own environment. Intervention is supplied according to need, not age or culture, although appropriate attitudes to specific client groups and the necessary knowledge of social considerations is essential. Physiotherapists specialising in rehabilitation of older people are trained to consider support systems, housing, available help and motivation. Rehabilitation of ethnic minority elders should not be considered a special problem, but an area of work requiring additional skills.

The aim of physiotherapy with elderly people is realistically to assess the patient and his or her surroundings and carers, and then plan a programme of rehabilitation to achieve goals agreed between all parties. In some cases, deterioration in the patient's condition may be inevitable due to the disease process. If this is the case, physiotherapy intervention can be considered to prevent complications, or stated as not able to help and be sensitively withdrawn (Squires and Wardle, 1988).

Rehabilitation of the elderly is by necessity a team effort, and in considering the views of 'all parties', the views of the various members of the team must be elicited. Team members may come from many cultures and their attitudes to rehabilitation may differ and must be considered in the goal setting process.

To achieve quality care, the physiotherapist will be concerned with:

- the range of disabilities or disadvantages suffered by respective groups;
- the level of expectation each group member brings with them;
- the level of participation that each individual and his/her carer is able – or prepared – to provide in the treatment process (Williams, 1979).

This is achieved by the process of clinical decision analysis which provides a system of assessment, goal setting, appropriate intervention and review.

Assessment

The purpose of assessment has been described by Rubenstein (1983) as to provide a diagnosis, plan for therapy and services, consider appropriate placement and provide a baseline against which change can be monitored. It should be noted that 'change' is the key word as conditions can change in either direction, but treatment should be effective against set goals; for instance a dying patient can still be treated with dignity and prevented from developing pressure areas, contractures and a chest infection.

The process of physiotherapy assessment of the elderly patient, together with documentation and evaluation, have been fully described elsewhere where the conclusion was drawn that locally agreed systems improve compliance so long as all the relevant components are included (Squires, 1986). These will depend on the membership of the team and allocation of responsibility. Multidisciplinary assessment and evaluation, although complex, can be efficient, informative and essential in the process of audit.

It should be remembered that diseases of the past in Britain, such as polio or tuberculosis, on which the current problem may be superimposed, may be little known except in theory to the newly qualified physiotherapist and may require additional research. In addition, the current problem may be previously unknown to the patient, such as stroke in cultures with a low life expectancy, and explanation and prognosis may be necessary.

The aim of the assessment is to define the actual problem, its prognosis and its effect on the individual's lifestyle.

Home assessment

At this stage, if the patient is an in-patient, or only seen at the day hospital or other venue away from home, an assessment of the home situation is essential. This should be undertaken by members of the team relevant to the situation with appropriate joint discussion beforehand and afterwards. The purpose of the assessment will be to appreciate the pattern of life that the patient will wish to return to, and the availability of support systems. The long and short term goals, together with the treatment plan, will be formulated in response to these observations and in discussion with patient, carer and colleagues.

Goal setting and evaluation

Once the findings of the assessment process have been identified, goals can be set which must be understood and agreed to voluntarily by the patient, carers and other team members. It should be remembered that goals are for the benefit of the patient and his or her carer. Lack of agreement with the goals planned by the therapist must be respected, and aims reconsidered, otherwise frustration affecting both parties and non-compliance by the patient will result. From the patient's point of view this will lead to a less than satisfactory outcome, and from the therapist's perception to lack of job satisfaction and its effect on morale and recruitment.

When setting goals with elderly people the habits of a lifetime must be considered – after 80 years a patient may be neither willing nor able to change the way he or she sits down, even if a very good reason is given. Practice may break a habit, but give and take and acceptance of a situation if it is safe may have to be tolerated although 'not by the book' and abhorrent to the perfectionist! If a habit has to be broken, then consistency from the team and carers is essential. Goals must also include the realistic capacity of the patient and carer – it has been noted in a simple grip test project that there are differences in muscular power between cultural groups, and this may have goal setting implications.

Short and long term goals should be agreed by the patient, carer and all members of the multidisciplinary team and should be set so that the eventual aim is known, and the components can be observed with consequent satisfaction for all concerned as they are achieved. Documentation that demonstrates visually the desired goals and progress will not only ease communication where language may be a barrier, but will be a source of feedback and stimulation. Such an example, where all patients referred to physiotherapy were assessed for their current level of performance and the mutually ageed goals were set, is given in Fig. 13.1. All team members as well as the patient and carers could then see change occurring. The criteria for each function were available to the assessors and evaluation of the outcomes can be measured.

Mobility index used for Physiotherapy assessment and evaluation

To be completed by the physiotherapist for each patient assessed   Patient's name ....

Level of independence	Prior mobility date				Initial assessment date				Aim of treatment				Pre-discharge assessment date		
	C	B	A		C	B	A		C	B	A		C	B	A
1. In / out of bed and bed mobility															
2. In / out chair															
3. Toilet															
4. Walks inside															
5. Stairs if necessary															
6. Up from floors															

Levels of independent performance:

C. Cannot do, does not do, or requires skilled help to perform activity
B. Needs some help, verbal or physical, to carry out activity
A. Independent, needs no help from another person, may use aids if required

From Squires *et al.* (1987). Reprinted by permission of the *Physiotherapy Journal*

Intervention

Once assessment and goal setting have identified the problem and goal to be achieved, the treatment plan can be devised using all the techniques available to the physiotherapist consistent with the established contraindications.

Where communication is a problem due to language difficulties, an interpreter at the assessment, goal setting and initial treatment stage is essential. The physiotherapist's skills in handling patients and eliciting neuromuscular responses such as when using weight bearing, ice, heat, PNF and Bobath techniques will be communication itself. The facilitation of movement is designed for the minimal use of words, as can be seen effectively in paediatrics. This has been transposed into use with elderly confused people by Oddy (1987) where facilitation through handling, provision of suitable furniture and repetition was shown to elicit the desired response. The practical nature of the treatment plan will also mean that the physiotherapist can demonstrate to the patient what he or she is required to do and encourage practice. Feedback can be given without the need for language, but it must be appreciated that cultural contexts differ; for example a pat on the back can be seen in some cultures as praise and in some as a rebuke.

As good handling can elicit the desired response, so poor handling can elicit the opposite and team members will need instruction in handling skills which they do not possess.

Practice of the skills learnt or re-learnt during treatment sessions is an essential component of most physiotherapy programmes, and these are frequently supplemented with handouts. In the case of non-English speaking/reading patients, such handouts will need translation and inclusion in the review and updating cycle.

Other considerations for physiotherapists

Views on disability and disfigurement in all cultures vary considerably – from being seen as the natural result of the disease process, to selection in response to past good or bad deeds. The desire to be treated in private should be respected.

Reactions to treatment by physiotherapeutic modalities are based on the physiotherapist's expectations from experience with patients. As in Britain to date the majority of patients are from the indigenous population, and studies on the reactions of different cultural groups are needed. For instance it is known that pain tolerance, bone density, and skin viability are largely racially determined physiological phenomena. Skin colour may obscure bruising, burns and gangrene. Attitudes to scarring when new tissue may differ in colour, and to amputation with alteration to body image, need consideration.

In terms of techniques, expectoration may be unacceptable to someone with experience of a country where tuberculosis is still prevalent and spitting an offence – much to the frustration of the therapist charged with obtaining a sputum specimen. In other cultures spitting may be seen as acceptable behaviour. Hydrotherapy may be unacceptable either through perceived hygiene considerations with the 'sharing of water', or through the exposure of the body to others in only a swimming costume. The latter has been overcome in some public baths either by special sessions, or by the wearing of light 'coverall' clothing.

Another factor worth considering is the provision of aids and appliances. Calipers and artificial limbs are now available to match skin colour, but surgical collars, splints and support stockings are generally only available in beige, white or pink. The provision of calipers requiring a supportive shoe may be a problem for those unused to heavy outdoor shoes such as the Chinese where light canvas shoes are the norm. Ankle orthoses may need to be of the moulded, insert type and a compromise reached on slightly stronger shoes. The clothing to be worn over the appliance may also require adaptation.

Many NHS walking aids and wheelchairs in the United Kingdom are re-conditioned and re-supplied. Experience of an insurance-based health care system may have led the patient to expect new and thus be highly offended by the appearance of 'second hand', acceptable only to those conditioned to a welfare system.

Mental illness

Physiotherapy in mental illness is a relatively new discipline and may confront the unwary with challenges not previously experienced. A particular problem in transcultural medicine can occur with elderly people with dementia from any culture. In such a situation, inhibitions may be lost and normally guarded comments expressed, often in explicit language and sometimes with violence. It has been shown (Denham, 1990) that 25 per cent of health and social services staff have suffered minor threat or abuse, the rate being higher in psychiatric hospitals. In working with such patients, most staff will have been at the receiving end of an offensive personal comment, but racially offensive remarks give the greatest resentment. An understanding of the cause, and empathy with the victim, whether staff or fellow patient, may help the situation. Also the families' reaction to the lack of inhibition may be one of embarrassment, and this needs a sympathetic approach.

Repatriation

The progress towards independence and the wish ultimately to return 'home' at the end of life may stimulate discussion with the therapist on the feasibility of such a new hope. Funding may be available and health requirements met, but all staff have a responsibility to ensure that patients are aware of the health care system they are returning to. Active rehabilitation may or may not be available, family support uncertain. An informed frank appraisal with the patient of the feasibility of returning may be less distressing than the reality.

Conclusion

Physiotherapy with any patient is dependent on co-operation which is elicited by understanding, empathy, respect, explanation, realistic assessment, joint goal setting, encouragement and feedback. With elderly people, social attitudes and health beliefs held by any culture must be understood to make the rehabilitation process work. Where the physiotherapist and patient are from different cultures these attitudes and beliefs must be appreciated by both so that the physiotherapy plan can respond to the needs of the patient. Such patients can be a source of such knowledge – if only we seek it.

References

DENHAM, M. (1990). Violence against health and social service staff. *Care of the Elderly*, **2** (4): pp. 139–40.

ODDY, R. (1987). Promoting mobility in patients with dementia: some suggested strategies for physiotherapists. *Physiotherapy Practice*, **3** (1): pp. 18–27.

PARRY, A. (1990). How do you think about physiotherapy? *Physiotherapy*, **76** (4): p. 197 RUBENSTEIN, L. (1983). The clinical effectiveness of multidimensional geriatric assessment. *Journal of the American Geriatric Society*, **31** (12): pp. 758–62.

RUBENSTEIN, L. (1983). The clinical effectiveness of multidimensional geriatric assessment. *Journal of the American Geriatric Society*, **31** (12): pp. 758–62.

SQUIRES, A. (1986). Physiotherapy assessment of the elderly patient. *Physiotherapy*, **72** (12): pp. 617–20.

SQUIRES, A. and WARDLE, P. (1988). To rehabilitate or not? In SQUIRES, A. (ed.) *Rehabilitation of the Older Patient*, pp. 102–22. Croom Helm, London.

SQUIRES, A., WILLIAMS, R., DOLBEAR, R. and SMOKER, S. (1987). Evaluation of physiotherapy in a day unit. *Physiotherapy*, **73** (11): pp. 596–8.

WILLIAMS, J. (1986). Physiotherapy is handling. *Physiotherapy*, **72** (2): pp. 66–70.

WILLIAMS, S. (1979). The quality of life of the elderly in ethnic minorities: the need for a new policy and strategy. In GLENDENNING, F. (ed.) *The Elders in Ethnic Minorities*. Beth Johnson Foundation, Stoke-on-Trent.

14

Occupational therapy with ethnic minority elders

Clephane A. Hume

Elderly members of ethnic minority groups face issues in addition to the general sociological problems and difficulties associated with ageing. Attention should be given to their special needs.

Possible problems have been detailed in earlier Chapters and some of these are particularly relevant to the occupational therapist. Such problems include deprivation in all its various aspects but, most noticeably, the loneliness consequent on separation as contact with the extended family is reduced or lost. Grandchildren may seem to be living in an alien world and the cultural distance of the intergenerational gap may be distressing.

Communication difficulties may increase as elderly friends and relatives die, and those who speak the mother tongue become fewer. This restricts social contact and ability to participate in decision making about different aspects of life. The person may feel alone, depressed and without a role or purpose in life.

In accordance with the code of professional conduct (1990) of the College of Occupational Therapists, occupational therapists are required to treat all patients according to their individual needs. The aim of the occupational therapist working with the elderly is to enable them to retain their independence for as long as possible. The problems resulting from physical and/or psychological illness are assessed and programmes of treatment are devised to maximise the use of the individual's abilities. Modifications to the environment may be necessary and attention will be given to the social context in which the person is living.

A variety of activities may be utilised in enabling elderly people to maintain or regain the ability to carry out their day to day tasks, to avoid dependency and to enjoy a satisfactory quality of life. Working within a multicultural setting can be challenging, but there are many rewards.

This chapter outlines some aspects to be considered when working with elderly people from different cultures.

Assessment and treatment planning

General considerations

Assessment forms the baseline from which to draw up a treatment programme. When working with ethnic elders, the therapist has a greater than usual need to be aware of the patient's social background in order to put his or her problems into context. Expecting a patient to carry out a task which is unacceptable to his or her

value system is not beneficial. Every effort should be made to a
caused by cultural misunderstanding. Contacts with the loc
knowledge of support structures available, will be valuable in r
back into the community.

In any initial assessment, the therapist seeks to identify
problems and general mental state, in order to distinguish
treatment from those of a more long term nature.

It should be remembered that admission may not be viewed
providing relief from the stress of illness, but rather may represe
the family, the principal source of support and communication.
considerations of the occupational therapist will be how to
communication.

What to assess?

Standardised assessment forms such as the Barthel Index or Crichto
may be completed, provided that the rater is aware of the degree of re ..... of the
items for any individual (Mahoney and Barthel, 1965). Individual occupational
therapy departments may have devised their own forms or rating schedules and
additional points may be added for particular ethnic groups.

Areas which the occupational therapist should consider include Activities of
Daily Living (ADL) with emphasis on personal care, domestic management and
community living skills. Interpersonal relationships and social activities will also be
relevant.

Additional data, such as information regarding place of birth and length of
residence in Britain, may be helpful if the person was not born here. Awareness
of the extent to which contacts exist beyond the immediate family and ethnic
group is also valuable. Such data must be sought tactfully in order not to create
offence.

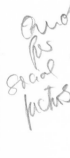

General considerations for treatment planning

"As occupational therapy is essentially a practically based profession which aims to
enhance patients' competence in daily living, it is important to be aware of social
roles and customs and how these will govern aims of treatment."

Expectations

Patients may expect staff to provide all the answers, often in the absence of much
information being volunteered. Clashes between expectations and treatment aims
are counterproductive and the therapist should make contact with the family to
ensure that decisions are made jointly, and the final aims understood by all.

Patients may, in their attempts to do what the therapist wishes them to, claim to be
able to undertake tasks which are unlikely to be within their capabilities. Reasons for
this may be complex. Perhaps to create an impression of not needing help – 'I can
cope' – to avoid loss of face, or simply as an attempt to please the therapist.

Loss of face

This is a concept which can be only partially understood by Western cultures who know what it is like to feel foolish through making a social gaffe or a public mistake. Loss of face goes much deeper than this; the individual's self esteem is ruined and his or her place in society may be lost. For an elderly person who should command respect, this may be particularly damaging. His or her total existence is threatened and sometimes suicide is seen to be the only acceptable response. The slur and stigma extend to the family and may create considerable social difficulties. Only tasks that can be assured of success may be attempted.

Responses of individuals to any apparent criticism may be coloured by attempts to avoid loss of face and this can be very exasperating for anyone who is unaware of the dynamics of the situation. It also has implications for psychiatry as difficulties are masked and any probing is firmly resisted. People may say 'yes' to avoid any suggestion of public disagreement or disrespect to the therapist.

The importance of religion

For many people, religion will be an integral part of day to day life. Respect should be accorded to religious practices such as specific times for prayer and the need to have significant objects to hand.

It is essential that the therapist is aware of any dietary restrictions before undertaking any cookery assessment or kitchen activities. These are described more fully in Chapters 7 and 17.

Family roles

Family structures may vary from the average British nuclear family to the extended kinship system in the context of which all decisions are made. The medical team may have to wait while overseas relations are consulted about the final stages of rehabilitation – not easy when there is pressure for rapid discharge.

The therapist should recognise that some of the attitudes found in Britain display what is regarded as shocking lack of respect for family values and responsibilities towards the elderly, and that this may cause offence to others. For example, the therapist may expect that a woman would be willing to assist her disabled father-in-law with tasks such as dressing. For an Indian, this would be disrespectful and therefore totally inappropriate.

Social roles

Social roles may be closely linked to religious and family customs as described above. The respect traditionally accorded to elders and the living arrangements of the extended family may have broken down, but certain role expectations remain. These include distinct divisions in sexual roles. A woman who has always maintained purdah (seclusion) will suffer extra problems when widowed and this may create practical difficulties if she has no male relatives who can undertake tasks such as shopping for her. Despite any individual feelings or values, it is not appropriate to impose one's own ideas of behaviour on women who belong to male dominated cultures. Equally, the man whose wife is disabled may have no experience of cooking and not regard this as his role.

In the context of disability which would suggest more equal sharing of roles, or even role reversal between husband and wife, the therapist must remember that this may be quite unsuitable. A female relative may be expected to take on the task as her recognised duty.

Individuality

The occupational therapist's aim is to restore the person to an optimum level of personal independence and quality of life. This varies between cultures, generations within cultures, and between individuals.

Introducing treatment and selection of media

When planning programmes for patients from a variety of ethnic backgrounds, the skills the occupational therapist requires will be unchanged. It is the application of those skills which varies, according to cultural needs.

For many patients, occupational therapy is an unknown concept and the focus on 'doing' may well be alien, especially for the elderly, who may enjoy 'watching the world go by', or participating in family affairs. What should the occupational therapist contribute? Is activity really appropriate?

In determining treatment goals, and selecting activities and media, there are various considerations to be made. These are described in general terms. A flexible approach is required.

Personal care

The obvious stumbling block here is male-female relationships and a sensitive awareness of this is required. In some cultures, a man may not discuss personal topics with a female therapist or vice versa. It is usually accepted that a male therapist will not undertake dressing practice with a female patient, but it should be recognised that for many elderly male patients, it is simply not appropriate to expect them to be assessed or treated by a female therapist. As already indicated, this would also apply on return home. On no account should such conventions be flouted.

Clothing styles should be considered and where disability makes dressing difficult, unless acceptable help is available, alternative methods should be devised in discussion with the patient. For example, if standing balance is a problem, it may be possible to teach a woman to put on her sari while sitting down. (Make the pleats in the centre and pin them in place. Wrap one end round the waist. Place the other over the shoulder and tuck in ends.) The most common Asian clothing styles are described to demonstrate the complexities involved.

Muslim women should traditionally be clothed from head to foot and their clothes should conceal the shape of their bodies. Muslim women from Pakistan and Gujarat traditionally wear kameez (tunic), shalwar (trousers) and dupatta or chuni (scarf). Muslim women from Bangladesh traditionally wear a sari with an underskirt and a waist-length blouse. The shalwar kameez or sari are usually worn as day and night wear but are loosened at night for comfort. Muslim women who wear Western dress will usually wear trousers or long skirts.

Most Muslim men wear Western style shirt and trousers. Traditional Pakistan male dress is kameez (shirt) and pajama (loose trousers). Bangladeshi traditional male dress is a shirt and a lungi, which is a length of cloth wrapped around the waist reaching down to the calves. Muslim men cover their heads with a brimless hat while praying.

The five signs of Sikhism and the turban have already been mentioned. The hair is allowed to grow and fixed in a bun (jura) on top of the head concealed under a turban. Most Sikh women wear shalwar kameez and the men tend to wear a Western style shirt and trousers.

Kaccha (special undershorts) may cause particular problems in hospital. Although traditional kaccha reached down to the knees, many Sikhs now wear ordinary underpants. However, they will have the same religious significance and devout Sikh men and women will never remove them completely: one leg is put it the new pair before the old pair is removed.

Most Hindu women wear a sari over a blouse and underskirt. Hindu women of Punjabi origin may wear a shalwar kameez instead of a sari. Most Hindu men wear Western style clothes, although some will wear traditional dress or a kameez (shirt) and pajama (trousers) at home.

If a woman has plaited hair, which is difficult to manage, a bun may be a possible alternative. She will be reluctant to have it cut and this is not a viable option. Likewise, a man may not be able to tie his turban but may be able to use one that is already made. Failing that, a woollen hat may be acceptable.

Personal hygiene in many cultures requires that people bathe in running water – a shower is used in preference to a bath. It may also be the practice to wash after using the toilet, rather than to use toilet paper. These points should be borne in mind when carrying out home visits.

The therapist should be aware of cultural practices regarding laterality. The left hand may be used for washing, the right for eating. This has obvious implications for the hemiplegic patient, which should be discussed sensitively.

Eating with the hand requires dexterity, holding a bowl near the mouth and using chopsticks may be no longer possible. A spoon may be an acceptable alternative.

Cooking and household management

Cooking may serve as an introduction both to therapy and to other patients. Multicultural cookery groups may provide social contact as well as being a way of practising skills and increasing self esteem.

Perhaps fresh food is purchased on a daily basis from the local market. Perhaps it is the man's role to do the shopping. Relatives should always be asked whether or not their family member will be expected to cook after returning home. Whatever the case, treatment should be geared towards accommodating the conventional pattern.

Lengthy procedures may be involved in preparing food and the use of assistive devices or methods of energy conservation may be appropriate in enabling a woman to retain her domestic status. Ability to make chapattis or to measure spices in the correct quantity may be an important aspect of daily life. Ascertaining safety, for instance in using a hot wok, may be necessary.

Distribution of meals throughout the day will follow differing patterns. The therapist should be aware of different dietary requirements and practices. A Muslim patient will not eat pork, and any other meat should be specially prepared (halal meat). Hindus are vegetarian and Orthodox Jews must keep a kosher kitchen. In carrying out cookery assessments, it may be relevant to remember that breakfast may not be tea, toast and cereal, but a bowl of soup and noodles. For Chinese people, rice is of prime importance and takes several forms.

Laundry and cleaning should also be considered and adaptations to methods devised where necessary.

Long term residence in Britain does not imply knowledge or acceptance of resources and entitlements to benefits which would be helpful in daily life. The therapist may provide relevant information or ensure that referrals to appropriate agencies are made.

Leisure   L + P.

Time may be passed in conversation with family and friends, rather than participating in activities outside the home. Growing old in another country may deprive many people of traditional social networks and familiar pastimes. When a sense of isolation is the major problem, identifying opportunities for unstructured social contact in the community is an important aspect of treatment. Local community centres may run special lunch clubs or friendship afternoons as described in Chapter 6.

Sharing of traditional art or music may lead to enrichment and greater understanding between cultures and thus be beneficially utilised. It is also important in evoking memories and encouraging healthy reminiscing (see Chapter 3 for a description of the use of reminiscence through drama).

Traditional crafts may be relevant as treatment media, but the therapist should remember that what is a leisure pursuit for one may have been work for another. The 'occupational' aspect may render crafts alien and unnecessary in the eyes of the patient, who sees old age as a time for reduced activity. Any hint of 'work' may be shameful for a woman. There may also be designated male and female divisions and these cannot be transgressed.

Group activities

Sensitivity is needed in respect of group activities. Social activities may not be acceptable or will be so only within selected groups. They may also prove to be highly enjoyable.

Selecting patients to participate in groups will be important in ensuring that all are able to contribute. This is perhaps most relevant in relation to reality orientation and reminiscence groups, where the inclusion of one, or a small number of ethnic minority members may create difficulties. Feelings of alienation may result if there is no shared background or a history of conflict between groups. Different memories can of course be used beneficially in extending the awareness of the group. Content of the reality orientation group must be sensitively chosen and relate to the culture and knowledge of the participants.

Individual and group activities require careful balance and should be selected according to the patient's needs at any particular time.

Home visits and community care

Home visits are undertaken routinely in order to assess the support available and the individual's ability to cope after leaving hospital.

As indicated above, there are various points to be borne in mind in being sensitive to relatives' feelings. Rules of hospitality must also be remembered – rejection of the refreshment offered may be interpreted as an insult. Other conventions may be less obvious – it may be the role of the guest to open the door on departure to avoid any implication of someone being hastened out. Conversations in the hall can be protracted if this is not understood.

Requirements for assistive devices have been briefly mentioned above in connection with selected problems. Adaptations will vary according to cultural practice and the options should be discussed with all concerned. Modesty must be respected and preserved. Suggestions for support services should be tactful, with careful explanations of the roles of different workers. To have a stranger as a home help may be unacceptable but volunteer visitors from community groups may be welcomed. Meals on wheels may be regarded as insipid, not prepared in accordance with religious requirements and consequently inedible.

Day care

Minority groups should, as their right, be asked to contribute to the planning of resources. While local amenities may include a mosque or temple, which can serve as a base for day care, facilities should be provided by the State rather than leaving the group to organise its own services in the absence of adequate provision. Some particular points should be taken into consideration.

- The number of day centres which cater for dietary needs is small. Failure to provide an acceptable meal may result in non-attendance.
- Specific programmes may be indicated, for example, the setting aside of a particular day for Asian clients attending a day centre.
- Separate male and female groups may also be necessary.

Psychiatric problems

Dilemmas in diagnosis

Dilemmas based on misunderstanding will inevitably occur. Lack of differentiation and nuances in language in respect of emotions may create blocks to communication. Literal translations or attempts at sign language may be highly misleading. Rack (1982) describes cultural pitfalls in respect of different psychiatric diagnoses. The occupational therapist may obtain information or observe behaviour which suggests psychiatric problems, and it is therefore valuable to have an understanding of symptoms. Selected examples will illustrate some commonly encountered situations.

Some symptoms may be linked to recognisable precipitating factors which often relate to social circumstances.

Depression

Probably the most well documented example of how presentation of symptoms may vary from one culture to another is that of somatisation in depression. Instead of the agitated, perhaps tearful patient who voices feelings of unhappiness, delusions of worthlessness or guilt, the therapist may find a person with a headache or sore stomach, for which no physical cause can be identified. Rather than pressing the individual to discuss feelings, it may be possible to treat him or her in the knowledge that this is a recognised presentation of depression in people who have no language or concepts with which to describe it other than physical symptoms.

Neglect of social roles may also indicate depression although this may be difficult for the therapist to identify correctly. There may be no indication of altered mood in the patient's conversation. It may be necessary to rely on the observations of the family in identifying variations in affective illness.

Factors contributing to depression may include racism and feelings of loss, either for the homeland or for a loved one.

The influence of racism in depression is worthy of consideration. Fernando (1986) has detailed the incidence of depression in ethnic minorities and explains very clearly the implications of racist attitudes for minority groups. He suggests that racism is more than an added stress. For someone who has spent many years in a foreign environment, the experience of alienation may damage self-esteem and create learned helplessness. An elderly person may have experienced the stress of moving to a new culture where attitudes towards incomers are not welcoming. Attempting to develop coping strategies and to improve self-esteem is to deal with only one side of the problem. We should also try to treat the cause.

Feelings of loss are widely acknowledged as contributing to depression and members of minority groups may have additional burdens in this respect. There may be a strong wish to return to the homeland, but the person realises that this would be impossible. Exiled friends may have managed to return, exacerbating the problem. Mourning for changes which have occurred in the homeland as the consequence of natural disasters or political events should also be acknowledged.

Bereavement is an obvious loss and here too there are added dimensions which may precipitate referral, for example, the Polish man whose Scottish wife dealt with day to day matters and shielded him from the difficulties resulting from his poor command of English. His understandable bereavement reaction was greatly magnified by his feelings of alienation. Similar situations are not uncommon in the case of Asian widows who have not learned to speak much English.

Organic illness: dementia

The incidence of dementia in many countries is lower than in the United Kingdom, largely due to shorter life expectancy. Assessment of dementia in immigrant members of the population may be more difficult because of communication problems. The elderly Eastern European lady who lost her command of English highlighted this. An interpreter was found and while her memory problems were not remediable, the situation was alleviated to some extent.

As with the other frailties of old age, confusion may be tolerated by the extended family and the person cared for without recourse to institutional care. When this is the case, relatives should be tactfully made aware of support services to which they are entitled if they so choose.

Conclusion

In essence, a high standard of professional practice, giving due attention to the needs of the individual, will serve the needs of ethnic minority elders.

This chapter has given some indications as to the variety and complexities of practice in a multicultural society and ways of promoting positive change have been indicated.

With a little judicious enquiry and willingness, the occupational therapist will gain a wealth of knowledge and experience the rewards of this area of work.

References

BRITISH ASSOCIATION OF OCCUPATIONAL THERAPISTS (1990). Code of Professional Conduct. *British Journal of Occupational Therapy*, 53 (4): pp. 143–8.

FERNANDO, S. (1986). Depression in ethnic minorities. In Cox, J. (ed.) *Transcultural Psychiatry*. Croom Helm, London.

MAHONEY, F. and BARTHEL, D. (1965). Functional evaluation: the Barthel Index. *Maryland State Medical Journal*, February.

RACK, P. (1982). *Race, Culture and Mental Disorder*. Tavistock Publications, London.

Further reading

BAVINGTON, J. and MAJID, A. (1986). Psychiatric services for ethnic minority groups. In Cox, J. (ed.) *Transcultural Psychiatry*. Croom Helm, London.

COX, J. L. (1986). (ed.) *Transcultural Psychiatry*. Croom Helm, London.

EDEN, S. (1987). Ethnic groups. In Bumphrey, E. (ed.) *Occupational Therapy in the Community*, pp. 221–2. Woodhead Faulkner, London.

GLENDENNING, F. (1979). *The Elders in Ethnic Minorities*. Beth Johnson Foundation Publications, Department of Adult Education University of Keele and Commission for Racial Equality, Keele.

HILL, C. (1986). Towards a better understanding of elderly migrants. *Australian Journal of Occupational Therapy*, 33 (2): pp. 71–6.

HUME, C. (1984). Transcultural aspects of psychiatric rehabilitation. *British Journal of Occupational Therapy*, 47 (12): pp. 373–5.

LIPSEDGE, M. and LITTLEWOOD, R. (1979). Transcultural psychiatry. In Granville-Grossman, K. (ed.) *Recent Advances in Clinical Psychiatry 3*. Churchill Livingstone, Edinburgh.

MARES, P., HENLEY, A. and BAXTER, C. (1985). *Health Care in Multiracial Britain*. Health Education Council and National Extension College Trust, Cambridge.

ORQUE, M., BLOCH, B. and MONROY, L. (1983). *Ethnic Nursing Care – a Multicultural Approach*. C. V. Mosby Co., New York.

SAMPSON, C. (1982). *The Neglected Ethic*. McGraw Hill, London.

15

Speech therapy with elderly people from linguistic minority communities

Deirdre M. Duncan

Speech and language problems in the elderly will include strokes and progressive illnesses as well as problems of communication which arise among the elderly from conditions of unknown or uncertain diagnosis, general deterioration and the ageing process. There is the important additional dimension for the elderly client from a linguistic minority community of having a different language and culture. Ironically, the client's main problem – a disorder in his or her home language – is the area which the therapist may be least able to access. This is the focus of this chapter.

The chapter presents a clinical perspective on the bilingual brain and considers the assessment and management of a range of acquired communication disorders. The general points made in Chapter 9 concerning enhancing communication, should be borne in mind throughout this chapter.

Being bilingual

Being bilingual means that a person has linguistic, communicative and sociocultural skills to varying degrees which allow him or her to perform in two (or more) linguistic communities. Hence, the bilingual person will be able to identify with the sociocultural features of the communities and become bicultural. Communicatively, a bilingual person should be able to behave appropriately at a nonverbal and pragmatic level in the two language communities. Linguistically, a bilingual person should be able to function in both languages, maybe not necessarily in literacy, and possibly not in identical situations but complementary ones. Some people, for example, may prefer to talk in English at work and about work, while using Urdu at home and at the Mosque.

In many cases, the elderly people in linguistic minority communities in Britain are not bilingual in the terms described above. They may have some English words and phrases but they function linguistically, communicatively and socioculturally as monolinguals in their home/community language.

The bilingual brain

The bilingual brain has developed the linguistic facilities to operate, that is understand and express, two or more languages. It is still a matter of controversy as to how the brain organises two or more language systems. The controversy revolves around whether the brain has distinct but related systems for each language or whether it has one language system operating different languages. In the event of neuronal deterioration or catastrophe, the pattern of language loss may reflect some of the bilingual neurolinguistic organisation.

There seems to be a tendency for the first, or home language to be the less impaired and to recover first (Pitre, in Albert and Obler, 1978). Also, remediation through one language system seems to trigger improvement in the other (Fredman, 1975). Further studies (Paradis *et al.*, 1982) have shown that immediately following a stroke in a bilingual person there may be a period of highly unstable interaction between the two languages, which will settle to a more stable pattern over a period of months. The implications are that clinicians may be best advised to wait six months post-trauma, as recommended with monolingual English stroke patients (David *et al.*, 1982), before initiating assessment.

The range of acquired communication disorders

The range of acquired speech and language disorders considered here are aphasia, dysarthria, laryngectomy and dementia.

Aphasia

Aphasia is the generic term describing a variety of language deficits resulting from trauma and damage, as in a stroke, to specific areas of the neurolinguistic network.

Assessment   There are very few formal assessments of aphasia in languages other than English. The *Battery of Aphasia Testing* (BAT) by Michel Paradis (1987) offers assessment of aphasia in 40 languages. This is a remarkable achievement. Unfortunately, its exhaustive series of subtests (200) makes it an unlikely clinical tool, at least in its entirety. A pithier aphasia assessment, albeit at screening level and in Punjabi and English only, is the *Panjabi Adaptation of the Aphasia Screening Test (Whurr)* by Kathryn Mumby (1988). It is best administered by a trained Punjabi/English bilingual co-worker. It provides clinically useful indications about the client's bilingual language profile which highlight areas for further assessment or therapy.

Management   In cases where the linguistic minority elderly client and the therapist share the minority language, or where there is a trained bilingual co-worker available, then therapy could progress in the minority language. It may be possible for the pre-morbidly bilingual client and the therapist to work through English, even when the speech therapist does not share the client's other (home) language. Therapy in English may trigger improvement in the client's other language. In such cases, clinicians should be aware that they will not be able to control or monitor the rehabilitation of the home language. This may cause the client and family some frustration and the therapist may have to arrange some way of managing this; for example through counselling the client and family or involving a bilingual co-worker when possible.

There is a wider discussion of assessment and therapy issues later in this chapter.

Dysarthria

Many progressive illnesses may lead to speech, language and/or swallowing disorders. Parkinson's disease, multiple sclerosis and motor neurone disease have a more frequent incidence, and Friedrich's ataxia, muscular dystrophy, myasthenia gravis and Huntington's disease are less frequent. The muscular problems caused by these illnesses effect the articulation of the organs involved in speaking and voicing (dysarthria), and swallowing (dysphagia).

Assessment   Assessing dysarthric speech must cover two areas. One area can assess the motor and sensory functions in non-linguistic framework and the other assess the articulations for the phonetic/phonology system which are language specific. Although the first area of assessment might be possible in theory without a bilingual co-worker, there may be some distress involved, particularly with an elderly client who neither speaks nor understands much English. In the case of a client who was pre-morbidly bilingual and has retained some English, or if the clinician shares the client's home language, then a bilingual co-worker may not be necessary at this stage. When assessing the language specific articulations, clinicians who do not share their client's language(s) will need a bilingual co-worker whose training has included ear training in articulation and voice for that language (for example tonal changes, retroflexion). In the case of pre-morbidly bilingual clients with a 'foreign accent', possibly because they acquired English in adulthood or overseas in their education, the challenge for the therapist will be to describe a target articulation pattern for the client in line with their pre-morbid performance. In the likelihood of not achieving this description, then the clinician may have to work towards a Standard English pattern which may present other difficulties.

The clinician may investigate the appropriateness of using one of the published dysarthria assessments, for example The Frenchay Dysarthria Assessment (Enderby, 1983), or modifying them, with the authors' permission, to include all the articulatory movements of the client's home language. Alternatively, informal assessment may yield the necessary information.

Assessment of dysphagia in the elderly linguistic minority client could be conducted by the clinician without linguistic complications. However, as noted above, the client may be very distressed by the swallowing disorder and, in the case where there is no shared language, the clinician may require the assistance of a trained bilingual co-worker to explain the disorder and counsel the client and if necessary the family.

Management   In dysarthria therapy there may be a certain amount that the clinician is able to do in a non-linguistic framework, such as breathing, voicing. However, unless the client was pre-morbidly bilingual and therapy can be done through English, therapy will be constrained without trained bilingual assistance. More important is that in speech and language disorders resulting from progressive illnesses, the clinician must be mindful of offering and training the client to use some effective form of communication as their illness progresses and their speech and language deteriorate. Advances are being made in high-tech communication aids which are appropriate for some linguistic minority clients. There may be difficulty in obtaining electronic aids in appropriate languages, voicing and scripts but advances are being made. Low-tech alternatives have been discussed in Chapter 9.

Counselling the client and family in their preferred language is essential. If this language is not English then a trained bilingual co-worker is imperative, unless the clinician shares the language. Every effort should be made so that the elderly linguistic minority client and their family understand the nature and the progress of the illness and the necessary changes along the communication spectrum from speech to communication aid.

Laryngectomy

The surgical operation to remove all or part of the larynx because of malignancy is called a laryngectomy. It results in aphonia and therapy aims to develop alternative voicing techniques.

Management   Speech therapy management must begin with pre-operative counselling, including an explanation of the operation and its implications on communication for the client. In the case of the elderly linguistic minority client, counselling must be in the language of their choice, which may be English if they are bilingual or in the home language. In the latter choice a bilingual co-worker will be needed. It is also good practice to arrange for a person of the same linguistic minority, who has had a successful laryngectomy, to visit the client pre-operatively. In the case where therapy can be conducted in English, the bilingual client may be able to generalise the alternative voicing technique and use it for the home language. In cases where the client does not speak English, the assistance of a bilingual co-worker is required.

Dementia

Dementia is the gradual failure of the brain functioning, usually due to Alzheimer's disease or multi-infarcts. Usually, language is disturbed when the dementia has progressed through the early stages. Semantic functions are the first language processes to be effected. In the later stages of dementia syntax and phonology are disturbed until, in severe dementia, the client may be able to communicate very little, possibly at the level of names only or less. Simultaneously, other brain functions are affected. These include memory, recall, and visual perception, all of which are important in language assessment and therapy. This pattern will obtain regardless of the client's language(s), although in the pre-morbidly bilingual client, the pattern of language disintegration may be complicated by the languages interacting.

Assessment   Aphasia assessments can be used to profile language modalities in dementia and, as studies have shown (Stevens, 1989), dementia language functioning may yield a differentially diagnostic profile. It may be appropriate to use the Punjabi adaptation of the AST(Whurr) (Mumby, 1988) in a similar way. The important factor about dementia is that visual perception is increasingly disturbed, which has implications for picture/object based assessment and therapy. If the elderly linguistic minority client with dementia were pre-morbidly bilingual, then in the early stages of language disturbance he or she might be able to cope with two culturally and linguistically diverse assessments. As the dementia progresses the ability to cope will deteriorate. In the case of the bilingual, we do not know how the two languages will deteriorate. It may be at different rates across linguistic levels and possibly dependent on many factors, such as pre-morbid use, context and materials stimulating retrieval. Much more research is needed to describe accurately the patterns of language disintegration in the bilingual client with dementia.

Therapy There are therapy programmes for people with dementia which are interdisciplinary and may involve the speech therapist, for example Reality Orientation (Holden and Woods, 1982). Such programmes are developed to stimulate and aid memory by encouraging recall of common experiences, such as the client's life during the last World War, or the coronation of Elizabeth II. They employ memory aids, such as photographs and objects, and orientation is inevitably towards clients who are English-speaking with a British cultural background. These programmes would not be immediately appropriate for ethnic minority people with dementia. It might be possible to develop a similar programme for a minority language and culture but, although this would involve considerable planning, time and resources, a start has been made by the Age Exchange Theatre Trust (*see* Chapter 3). In districts with large populations of an ethno-linguistic minority, this type of investment should be carefully considered with a view to making a package available to districts with smaller, similar population groups.

Hearing impairment

Hearing impairment may complicate all the above mentioned communication disorders or it may appear alone as a result of trauma, industrial environment or part of the ageing process. Although it may not necessarily effect the client's speech and language, loss of hearing can cause problems in communication with others, along with a great deal of frustration, anxiety and isolation. It is not always easy to detect prior to referral and investigation. Raising awareness about hearing impairment in the elderly through health education may be one way forward. Conducting the audiology investigation with an elderly linguistic minority client may require the assistance of a bilingual co-worker, and his or her further assistance may be required in counselling about the need to wear a hearing aid.

The remainder of the chapter will deal with the important features of case history taking, assessment, counselling and therapy as well as discussing the key role of the bilingual co-worker in speech therapy with the ethnic and linguistic minority client.

Case history taking

The case history of an elderly person referred with an alleged speech and language disorder must include information about medical, family and social history. In the case of the elderly client from a linguistic minority community, further information must be obtained about pre-morbid languages and the modes and patterns of use. It is important to develop a checklist of questions, such as what languages were spoken by the client, when each was last spoken and with whom, which languages were spoken by the client in a set of specific situations pertinent to the client – at home, at work, to children, to grandchildren, in friends' houses, in what languages did the client read and write, what about, to whom and when was the last time. This information will provide a pattern of sociolinguistic information, highlighting the range and modality of language(s) used and the situations and frequency of their use. A further two points concerning language status and scripts are worth bearing in mind. In some countries there are languages or dialects in which the education is conducted and these languages/dialects acquire higher status than the other languages/dialects in the country. For example, Urdu is a more prestigious language than Punjabi among Pakistani people, and Standard Italian is more prestigious than the 'dialetti' amongst Italians. There may be many socio-political factors encouraging the identification with one language/dialect group, even though it may not be the one spoken by the client. Consequently, it is important to identify accurately the spoken language or dialect of the client. In the assessment of literacy it will be useful if the clinician can recognise the different scripts associated with the different languages and communities. For example, Hindi is written in Devanagri script, Sikh-Punjabi in Gurmukhi script, Russian in the Cyrillic script, as well as the other languages which have their own scripts.

Assessment

Certain important principles should be practiced when using formal assessments to assess the English or elderly bilingual clients from ethnic or linguistic minority communities. Just as when using monolingual English assessments for developmental language disorders, great care must be taken when interpreting the results from bilingual adults. Any comparison of disturbed speech and language patterns in English from a bilingual with patterns derived from monolingual English speakers can only be done at a descriptive level (Grosjean, 1989). The clinician should be aware that English (British, United States, Canadian or Australian) formal language assessments may present additional cultural problems for the elderly client from an ethnic or linguistic minority community, which may be aggravated by visual perception problems.

Any attempt to 'transfer' an English language assessment into another language requires serious study in order to be successful. A good example is Mumby's (1988) work. Such a study must consider the appropriate grammatical structures and vocabulary of the target language, the stimuli across modes, accomodating writing scripts and making the materials age and culture appropriate. Moreover, this type of study must be taken up if speech and language assessments are to become available in languages other than English in order to assess non-English speech and language disturbance. Speech and language assessments in other languages need not be based on an English equivalents, although in the first instance it may help.

Informal assessment of speech and language disorder can be most successfully carried out when the speech therapist shares the minority language of the client. When the client's minority language is not shared by the clinician, certain basic resources need to be in place. The clinician should be familiar with the structure of the minority language through grammar books and dictionaries and there should also be personnel who share the minority language of the client – preferably a trained bilingual co-worker. A 'helper', such as an interpreter, relative or friend may be an alternative, albeit a less satisfactory one.

Initially, the clinician needs a corpus of the client's expressive language data to analyse and a 'helper' can clearly help to provide the data in the minority language by eliciting speech, language and other skills which can be tape recorded. It is unlikely that the 'helper' would be able to assist in the transcription and analysis of the data. A colleague in another district or an applied linguist who shares the client's minority language may be able to help. Subsequent detailed linguistic investigation and therapy may be constrained without substantial knowledge of the minority language on the part of the clinician.

The clinician and the co-worker must spend time developing a sufficient, basic bank of linguistic resources, such as word lists, minimal phonological pairs, semantic pairs, structures suitable for 'cueing', and materials, before initiating assessment and therapy. There may be outstanding linguistic information which cannot be prepared, such as word frequency lists, which may constrain assessment and therapy.

Finally, it is important to recognise that the assessment of the speech and language disturbance of the elderly ethno-linguistic client will take considerably longer than that of an English monolingual client even when there is a bilingual co-worker, or when the therapist shares the client's minority language(s).

Counselling

The principles of counselling obtain in the case of the ethnic and linguistic minority elderly client although they will need to be adapted and applied to different linguistic and cultural approaches. It is important that clinicians recognise their limitations in transcultural counselling skills and are prepared to train further and to work with trained bilingual co-workers and/or other transcultural professionals. In addition to offering an explanation of the disorder in terms that can be understood by the client/family, counselling may involve discussing the concept of 'rehabilitation' as compared with 'cure' and, in particular, the process of speech and language rehabilitation. It will involve helping the client and family to come to terms within their own cultural framework with the implications and consequences of the speech and language disturbance. Without transcultural skills or appropriate personnel counselling may not be possible.

Therapy

Language choice

A balanced clinical decision about language choice in therapy could be made if the necessary clinical infrastructure and linguistic information was in place and available; for example, bilingual speech therapists, trained bilingual co-workers, assessments in other languages, linguistic information about other languages, pre-morbid sociolinguistic information about the client, a speech and language profile in the client's languages. Where there is little infrastructure, it will be difficult to obtain linguistic profiles of the client's skills and the clinician must make clinical compromises such as working through English, a language only partly shared by the client. In the case where the elderly client is monolingual in a minority language, every effort should be made to offer assessment and management in that language. In the case of lack of resources, the clinician feels unable to initiate the rehabilitation process and must be sure that the management and planning levels of the service are aware of the decision and the reasons for it.

A decision to initiate the rehabilitation process in English with the monolingual minority language client may have a negative effect on the elderly client, possibly resulting in self-discharge. Alternatively, the elderly client and family may respond positively to therapy in English, interpreting it as a means of learning a 'high status' language.

The language repertoire of the elderly linguistic minority client before and after the start of the language disturbance will influence choice of therapy language. The language preference of the client and family should be canvassed as another factor in deciding on the language for therapy.

Language therapy techniques

The strategies which are employed by clinicians in therapy at different levels of lanaguage breakdown – phonology, syntax, semantics – are based on the structure and function of English. When working in another language these strategies have to be amended and adapted to the different linguistic structures of the language and their functional appropriateness. For example, build-up cues in English which may be designed to elicit vocabulary or to establish functional phrases would not achieve the same structural objective in another language, such as Punjabi, which has a subject-object-verb (SOV) structure.

Example 1: 'fish and . . .' (chips)
This is not a functionally appropriate cue for many North and South Asian clients who do not eat fish and chips.

Example 2: 'drive the . . .' (car)
This is not a linguistically appropriate cue for SOV languages where the cue would need to be structured to elicit 'drive', the verb,
– 'car . . .' (drive)
The context of the cue would need to have been set so that the verb inflections – the past/present tenses, gender, case and number agreement – would be controlled and part of the objective.

Some assessment and therapy techniques involve working with visual materials which may be one of the client's strengths. Bearing in mind the high level of per-morbid illiteracy in elderly linguistic minority clients, extending visual/oral strategies into the written mode may not be possible. This may have a constraining effect on therapy strategies and on general communication.

The importance of culturally-appropriate materials cannot be over emphasised. Materials which are user-friendly encourage the client to identify with the rehabilitation process and stimulate the desire to communicate. It will prevent confusion on the part of the client about what is expected of him or her. For example, in an expressive language activity to stimulate the description of a sequence of events, there might be a sequence of pictures depicting a woman making a cup of tea: filling the kettle with water from the tap, putting tea in to the pot, adding the boiling water to it, pouring it in to the cup and adding milk and sugar. While making a great deal of sense to someone from English culture, this would be almost meaningless to people from other cultures who may not drink tea or, if they do, would not make it like that. By visiting multicultural bookshops and stores, clinicians can equip themselves with a range of materials suitable or adaptable for therapy purposes.

The bilingual co-worker

Throughout this chapter the role of the bilingual and bicultural co-worker has been highlighted as being essential to the rehabilitation process in many cases of speech and language disorder in the elderly linguistic minority client. The co-worker facilitates the speech therapist's work in the client's minority language not shared by the therapist. Thus the co-worker is instrumental in developing a good rapport with the client as well as enabling counselling, case history taking, assessment and therapy. The co-worker provides the clinician with the crucial language and cultural skills to access the client's minority language repertoire.

Recruitment of a bilingual co-worker should reflect the demographic needs of the linguistic minority communities in the district, specifically in language. Country of origin, culture, religion and gender may also need to be considered. It may follow that a number of co-workers are required.

Optimum clinical practice can be achieved when suitable training is offered to the co-worker. It must include linguistic analysis of the co-worker's minority language, counselling skills and confidentiality, test administration and ear-training, as a basis which can be developed according to the needs of the caseload. There must be a 'good working relationship' between the therapist and co-worker, that is, an appreciation of each other's roles and each other's skills. However, the speech therapist must always carry the caseload responsibility. Details about working with bilingual co-workers can be found elsewhere (Barnett, 1989).

In the case of the linguistic minority client when there is no trained bilingual co-worker available, the alternatives which the clinician may seek, such as working with an interpreter, a relative or a friend of the client, will take the clinician further away from the likelihood of achieving an accurate linguistic assessment, providing transcultural counselling or working through a therapy programme in the client's minority, and possibly only, language.

Conclusions

It is important that the clinician establishes the pre-morbid linguistic repertoire of the linguistic minority elderly client and is aware of the theoretical possibilities of interactions between the bilingual client's languages resulting from the disorder. Clinicians should familiarise themselves with the main minority languages in the district/caseload, in terms of language structure and basic vocabulary as well as culture. They should identify areas of further training, such as transcultural counselling. They should also identify and try to build up resources appropriate for this population group.

Finally, the management and planning levels of the speech therapy service should develop an appropriate infrastructure to meet the needs of the elderly linguistic minority client, for example by encouraging more linguistic minority speakers to train as speech therapists, recruiting more bilingual co-workers and initiating projects to develop assessments and therapy programmes in minority languages for dementia, aphasia and dysarthria.

References

ALBERT, M. and OBLER, L. (1978). *The Bilingual Brain*. Academic Press, New York.

BARNETT, S. (1989). Working with interpreters. In Duncan, D. (ed.) *Working with Bilingual Language Disability*. Chapman and Hall, London.

DAVID, R., ENDERBY, P. and BAINTON, D. (1982). Treatment of acquired aphasia: speech therapists and volunteers compared. *Journal of Neurology, Neurosurgery and Psychiatry*, 45: 957–61.

ENDERBY, P. (1983). *Frenchay Dysarthria Assessment*. College Hill, CA.

FREDMAN, M. (1975). The effect of therapy given in Hebrew on the home language of the bilingual or polyglot adult aphasic in Israel. *British Journal of Disorders of Communication*, 10: pp. 61–9.

GROSJEAN, F. (1989). 'Neurolinguists beware! The bilingual is not two monolinguals in one person. *Brain and Language*, 36 (1): pp. 3–15.

HOLDEN, U.P. and WOODS, R. T. (1982). *Reality Orientation*. Churchill Livingstone, Edinburgh.

MUMBY, K. (1988). An adaptation of the Aphasia Screening Test for use with Panjabi speakers. *British Journal of Disorders of Communication*, 23 (3): pp. 267–92.

PARADIS, M., GOLDBLUM, M-C. and ABIDI, R. (1982). Alternate antagonism with paradoxical translation behaviour in two bilingual aphasic patients. *Brain and Language*, 15 (1): pp. 55–9.

PARADIS, M., LIBBEN, G. and HAMMEL, K. (1987). *The Bilingual Aphasia Test*. Erlbaum, Hillsdale, NJ.

STEVENS, S.J. (1989). Differential naming difficulties in elderly dysphasic subjects and subjects with senile dementia of the Alzheimer type. *British Journal of Disorders of Communication*, 24 (1): pp. 77–92.

16

Chiropody and the ethnic minority elder: A study of take up and use of a service within a defined population

Seema Padhiar and Charon Bansal

Having defined the local population, the question of how to tackle the needs and demands of ethnic minority elders in Britain can best be answered by action. One must first assess the needs presented by this group and then look at how to meet their demands. The most appropriate and sensitive measure of any consumer need is research. The results derived are important in influencing any future strategy of an organisation, and this is equally applicable to a service such as chiropody. It is essential to recognise the needs of its target groups and to deliver the appropriate service.

This leads to the question of whether a service like chiropody in any Health Authority is aware of the issues and the special considerations related to ethnic minority groups, and especially to the elderly members, within its population.

To try and answer the above for Newham Health Authority, the district chiropody service carried out a pilot survey to 'identify' and record the number of ethnic minority patients treated by the department over a one month period. Newham has a population of 210 000 and the age groups, by birthplace of head of household, is shown in Table 16.1.

The elderly population can be seen to be made up predominantly by indigenous elderly. Figures for the 1981 Census are given in Table 16.2.

The main objective of the study was to try to identify the relative uptake of chiropody by minority groups and the likely pathology presented. It was envisaged that the results would underline any necessary recommendations in the area of service delivery. Another objective of the study was to make comparisons with other research findings. This proved difficult due to the lack of published data on the subject. It was noted that numerous publications existed concerning the subject of ageing in modern societies, but only a small proportion of those dealt with issues of ethnic minorities and health service availability and use. Even those that did recognise the problem did not discuss specifically the subject of ethnic minority elders and chiropody.

One piece of research (Donaldson, 1986) was invaluable in compiling this work. The information discussed is heavily reliant on this particular piece of work as no other relevant data was available. Constant comparison is made of the results of this survey with our own pilot study throughout the chapter.

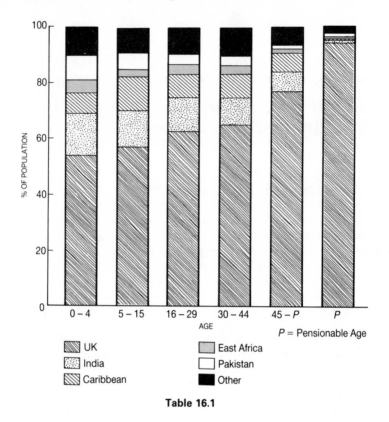

Table 16.1

Table 16.2   Composition by origin of the elderly population, as indicated by 1981 Census figures.

Origin	% of total
Indigenous	95
Indian	1
Caribbean	0.5
East African	1
Pakistani	0.5
Other	2

The pilot study

The study set out to identify and record the number of ethnic minority patients within the chiropody service in Newham Health Authority. It was decided to conduct the study by measuring the throughput of ethnic minority patients over a period of one month at a central clinic. The clinic was one that employed the widest variety of clinical treatments and thereby captured a good cross section of the different age groups and different pathologies presented.

Data collection

With the patients' consent (all consented), information was recorded in terms of age, sex, country of origin, medical status, and presenting pathology. This combination of variables allowed analysis for projecting present and future trends against the indigenous population and that of the ethnic group surveyed. The size of the sample did not allow significance testing but the findings led to the formation of recommendations.

In this way it was possible to observe the variety of pathology and to formulate a care package for the future consisting of appropriate advice, education, and treatment, with the emphasis always on prevention.

Table 16.3 Numbers of patients seen (all ages)

Age group	Ethnic minority population (actual no.)	(%)	Indigenous population (actual no.)	(%)
< 65 years	25	72	106	21
65–74 years	7	20	163	32
75–84 years	3	8	181	35
85 + years	0	0	62	12
TOTAL	35	100	512	100

Total number of patients seen:	547	
Total number of elderly (65+ years):	416	
Ratio of males: females		
– Ethnic minority population	1:1	
– Indigenous population	1:4	
Medical status (recorded as diabetic or non-diabetic		
– Ethnic minority population	70% diabetic	
– Indigenous population	10% diabetic	

Details of all the patients seen are given in Table 16.3. Over a one month period, 416 patients aged 65 or above were seen by the chiropody service. Of these 97.6 per cent were from the indigenous population and 2.4 per cent from the ethnic minority population.

As has already been identified, 95 per cent of the total population (all ages) is from the indigenous population and 5 per cent from the ethnic minorities. This shows that ethnic minority elders are under represented among the patients seen. The figures in Table 16.3 show that ethnic minority patients are heavily represented under 65, which can be explained by the fact that the majority of ethnic patients seen in this group were children. In the 65 – plus age group its decrease is 10 years behind the indigenous population, reflecting the age profile of the two different groups.

Another interesting factor is the ratio of males to females. In the ethnic minority population, this was 1:1, but in the indigenous population it was 1:4. This again reflects the age profile, with indigenous female elderly outliving males.

The medical status of patients showed that 70 per cent of ethnic minority elders were diabetic, compared with 10 per cent of indigenous elders (rough figures only), and this is in line with the estimates in Chapter 8 of South Asians having an incidence of diabetes five times that of the indigenous population.

The presenting pathology (interpreted by type of clinic attended) is outlined in Table 16.4. The higher incidence of nail surgery and re-dressing probably reflects the higher rate of diabetes in ethnic minority elders.

Table 16.4 Presenting pathology

Clinic attended	Ethnic minority elders (%)	Indigenous elders (%)
Routine clinic	70	88
Nail surgery	10	1.5
Re-dressing clinic	20	10.5

Interpretation of findings

Before drawing any inferences or making any comparative analysis it would be apt to re-emphasise the heavy reliance upon Donaldson's paper. Constant comparison is made between this and our findings. From the findings it is possible to highlight a number of interesting presentations including those of clinical value.

From the figures it can be seen that there is a low uptake of chiropody by the ethnic minority population. Low uptake of the service can be attributed to various factors, most of these relating to cultural and traditional attitudes. The two most striking of these are the importance of the extended family in Asian communities and the high rate of illiteracy amongst this group, most particularly the elderly members. These factors are generally known to be associated with immigrant populations and are not exclusive to those residing in Newham. Our study probably indicates these factors play a role in the low uptake of the service. To enable comparison with Donaldson's study, which was based on elderly Asians, the Asian patients only will be considered.

Family structure Donaldson's study indicated that most Asian families were large (73 per cent had three or more living children) and most had at least one child living with them reflecting the multigenerational households in which they live. Ninety-two per cent of the respondent's in Donaldsons survey felt that 'the family' should look after old people. The traditional viewpoint can also be explained by the domestic role of older Asian women within the family and therefore providing support and help, most probably including foot care. The change in the tradition of the extended family amongst Asian people, which is also seen in non-Asian families, will lead to a decrease in dependence on the family and an increased reliance on community services. For future research it will be important to discover the family support available to those who *did* attend the clinics and to compare with what is known of the population as a whole.

Literacy The Newham study did not seek literacy, but Donaldson's study indicated that only 21 per cent could speak English (over half with difficulty), and 65 per cent could read it. When female respondents were selected from the sample, the ability to read was reduced to 27 per cent and two thirds were illiterate in all languages.

Climate of home country   As current ethnic minority elders were probably resident in their home country during their childhood, it is necessary to consider what the 'traditional' footwear would have been which may have been transferred with them. Footwear is worn to suit the climate, and in hot countries this is frequently sandals. The change to closed footwear may have brought about some pathologies. However the influence of footwear as an aetiology of foot pathology is uncertain and current research seems to indicate that footwear is less of a factor than has been thought. Studies have shown that unshod people can still develop conditions such as *hallux valgus* (Lam and Hodgson, 1958) but the incidence is much lower than in shod races.

Occupation   Occupations of ethnic minority elders may have been different in their country of origin to those undertaken in the United Kingdom. The link between occupation and foot pathology has to be investigated. The generation of women in the elderly age group (especially those of Asian origin) was largely domestic and as this will have probably been the case on transfer to the United Kingdom, foot pathology is unlikely to have been influenced.

Pathology   The prevalence of pathology affecting foot conditions in the group studied may reflect the lower uptake. Whilst no studies have looked specifically at foot conditions in ethnic minority elders, studies have shown that medical pathology varies with culture such as the fivefold increased susceptibility to Type II Diabetes Mellitus in Asian immigrants in Britain (Gale, 1987).

Discussion on the project

This pilot project has highlighted a low uptake of chiropody services by ethnic minority elders in one health district. The results have raised further questions – such as the climatic, occupational and pathological influences on foot disorders – which require further investigation. The findings can then be interpreted locally to reflect the constituents of the main cultural groups (Jerome, 1983).

The problem of knowledge and accessibility can be addressed locally whilst further investigations, perhaps on a national scale, are undertaken.

Donaldson's study showed that 88 per cent had not heard of chiropody, 3 per cent were receiving it and a further 18 per cent felt the need for it. Although the latter is consumer defined, only attendance at a clinic and assessment by the chiropodist will determine whether this is a need that requires to be met.

Action plan

The action plan requires a fundamental approach, mainly that of raising awareness and overcoming communication problems. In this way uptake of the service can be increased, and the needs of this particular group can then be met.

The issue of raising awareness can be tackled first of all by educating those offering the service into recognising the special needs of the ethnic minority group. This implies incorporating teaching of the customs and backgrounds of minority groups during the training of chiropodists. Certain customs may appear peculiar to those unaware of them, for instance the touching of a person's feet by another individual is perceived as a mark of respect in Asian culture. Usually this is performed by a daughter-in-law to her father or mother-in-law, or grandchild to grandparent, sometimes even child to parent. Otherwise handling of feet is not accepted. In fact, physical contact of any kind is refrained from, especially between males and females. This even includes the handshake, which is accepted as a polite gesture in British society.

Anxieties can be brought about by differences in culture and can deter an individual from obtaining help. A typical example of this can be shown by the fact that many Asian women refrain from physical examination because they are normally expected to have their limbs covered and revealing a naked part of their body can be frightening to them. This aspect should be considered during biomechanical examination where a patient is usually instructed to wear shorts.

Patient to practitioner communication can also pose problems. In some Asian communities women may be forbidden to speak to a man and will be accompanied by another person (usually the husband or father) who will speak for them.

At present the schools of chiropody in Britain, do not, as far as is known, account for any differentiation of the population as part as their formal syllabus or curriculum. Occasionally passing reference is made to racial factors affecting the prevalance of a certain pathology, for example in lobster claw deformity. The emphasis of education can also be directed towards 'in-house' training. Staff should be made aware of the special requirements and customs that may be necessary and need to be understood for the population they are working with.

Newham is fortunate in that it employs linkworkers if there are communication problems. Currently this service is underused by the Chiropody Department but this could be improved.

Raising awareness amongst ethnic minority groups incurs challenges of its own. As mentioned previously, the rate of literacy amongst these individuals is low, and highly significant when figures show that nearly two thirds of the female group studied were illiterate in *all* languages. The problem of literacy is a large one; careers information on chiropody is included in numerous books and directories but this type of information (a valuable method of public relations) is meaningless if it cannot be read or understood. Conventional measures in health education, such as posters and leaflets printed in several languages, are therefore inadequate. A more useful way of promoting health education would be through media such as radio (Asian language programmes are listened to by a high percentage of old people), and video. Ownership and rental of video recorders is high among the Asian community that watches Indian video films as a popular pastime. The production of a health education 'video' could be an informative and relatively inexpensive venture. Such videos could be easily shown in general practices, health centres, etc. Newham is fortunate in that over half its chiropodists are able to speak at least one Asian language and it is highly likely that a video along the lines mentioned above will be made. Working with other disciplines on such a project should be given serious consideration.

For those who are literate, conventional health education measures are adequate and should be promoted as much as possible and made more accessible in health centres, doctors' surgeries, hospitals, clinics, libraries etc. and other places used by the target population. Increasing awareness must also include the co-operation of other health disciplines – Donaldson's study showed that 92 per cent of Asian elders had seen their general practioners in the six months prior to date of interview. This is a high figure compared to that of the indigenous population. If this group has a high level contact with their family doctor, then it is logical to suppose that greater liaison with the general practitioner service is required in order to encourage referrals where appropriate.

Conclusion

From the points discussed it is obvious that room exists for improving access to chiropody for the ethnic minority elder and that this can only be accomplished by positive action on a multidisciplinary basis. Most of all, research is required on a national scale and over a greater period of time in order to obtain a more accurate picture of the situation of the ethnic minority elder.

Continuous assessment and application of the action plan needs to be augmented to eradicate the apparent discrepancy between demand and supply for chiropody.

Referring again to Donaldson's study: few elderly Asians were aware of services, particularly chiropody. Language excluded them and it was recommended that health education intiatives must be directed at these people and an attempt made to understand these cultural and language barriers.

References

DONALDON, L. J. (1986). Health and social status of elderly Asians: a community survey. *British Medical Journal*, 293: p. 1079.

JEROME (1983). *Ageing in Modern Society*. St Martin's Press.

GALE, E.A.N. (1987). Diabetes Mellitus and other disorders of metabolism. In Kumar, P. and Clark, M. (eds.) *Clinical Medicine*. pp. 744–79. Balliere Tindall, Eastbourne.

LAM, HODGSON, (1958). A comparison of foot forms amongst the non-shoe and shoe wearing Chinese population. *Journal of Bone and Joint Surgery*, 40 (a): pp. 1058–62.

17

Nutrition and dietetics

Kiran Shukla

Diets of people from minority groups

> Food and diet are more than a
> means or even of a way to health.
> They are a part of the total way
> of life and culture of a group.
> (Todhunter, 1965)

Cultures are never static, they evolve through history modified by each generation. Despite change and the variations within ethnic groups and between individual members of a group, cultural food habits do have a common identity.

The choice, preparation, and indeed, the eating of food are all deeply embedded in the cultures and religions of the world. The actual foods consumed by different populations depend largely on income, geographical areas and whether people are living in an urban or rural setting. Religion and superstition also have some influence. People's religion plays an important role in the adoption of certain restrictions in the diet.

Dietary habits of various groups

Hindus

Over 80 per cent of people living in India follow Hinduism. Hindus in Britain come from the Indian States of Gujarat and Punjab and from East Africa. Hindus preach the doctrine of non-violence against any living thing. Orthodox Hindus will not eat any meat, fish or eggs. Western cheese which is made with rennet and jellies made from animal gelatine are not acceptable either.

Cows are sacred in India, hence beef is not eaten by Hindus. Milk, butter and cheese are considered pure foods. Non vegetarian Hindus vary from the ones who eat only eggs or fish, to some Hindus who will eat meat, fish and eggs. Beef and its products are not eaten even by the less strict Hindus. Pork is considered to be unclean and not generally eaten.

A traditional Hindu vegetarian diet will consist of:

- dahl, which is a dish of lentils or beans (pulses);
- vegetable dishes;
- curd or yogurt;
- chapattis or rice as a staple.

The majority of Britain's Gujarati community are Hindus. Gujarati Hindus have rice with every meal. They may have chapattis or puri (deep fried). The chapattis used in the Gujarati household are very small in size. Each one is approximately equivalent to one small slice of wholemeal bread. Most of the dishes in a Gujarati meal are served at the same time. A variety of dishes with pickles, chappatis, rice and sweetmeats/dessert may be served on a large stainless steel plate called 'Thali'. Some restaurants serving Gujarati food have 'Thali' on their menu.

Traditionally, elderly Hindus withdraw from the concerns of daily life and concentrate on praying and spiritual matters. They are careful about what they eat, hence eat only foods that are considered pure like milk, ghee, yogurt, nuts and fresh fruit. Some Hindus fast on various days. These fasts can be weekly, fortnightly, or monthly on special occasions. Usually, pure foods like milk, fruits and/or vegetables like potato, yam and sweet potato are allowed during the fast.

Some Hindus are followers of Swami-narayan. They do not eat onion and garlic which are considered undesirable stimulants.

Islam/Moslem religion

The majority of followers of Islam in Britain are from Pakistan, Bangladesh and East Africa. Moslems follow dietary laws laid down by the Qu'ran (Holy Book).

Dietary restrictions include the following.

- Eating of pork or pork products like sausages, bacon, ham or anything made with lard is forbidden.
- Meat should be slaughtered according to Islamic law. The animal is slaughtered by cutting the jugular vein and is dedicated to God by saying a short prayer which renders the meat 'Halal', hence meat sold in most British shops is not acceptable. Most Moslems take great care not to break food prohibitions and will not eat any food if they are not sure of the ingredients. Some very strict Moslems will only use Halal bread, biscuits etc. When eating outside in institutions, some Moslems prefer to call themselves vegetarians but accept eggs and fish.
- From adolescence to old age, Moslems are expected to observe a month long fast of Ramadan, which usually falls on the ninth month of the lunar year. During Ramadan, no food or beverage is consumed from dawn to sunset.

All Moslems are non-vegetarians. A traditional meal consists of meat or fish dish with chapattis or rice. People from Pakistan have wheat as staple and Bangladeshi's have rice as staple.

Sikhism

This is a fairly new religion which is an offshoot of Hinduism. It was founded in the 16th century by Guru Nanak. The majority of Sikhs are from the Punjab in North India.

Some Sikhs follow dietary restrictions similar to those of strict Hindus, hence are vegetarians. Generally, as a group, they are less strict. The non-vegetarian Sikhs eat meat which has been killed with one blow. Most of them do not eat beef or pork.

Most Sikhs will accept food cooked by other people as long as it conforms with the religious restrictions and is acceptable in terms of taste. Every Sikh temple (Gurdwara) has a communal kitchen in which food is cooked for the whole community at least once a week. This food is then eaten by the Sikhs after the prayers. Although Sikhism does not dictate vegetarianism, meat, fish or eggs are never served at the Sikh temple to avoid offending vegetarian Sikhs.

A traditional meal in a Sikh household is somewhat similar to a traditional Hindu vegetarian meal. The main differences are as follows:

- Most of the Sikhs have chapattis as a staple, rather than rice;
- Non vegetarians may replace dahl with a meat dish or have a meat dish in addition to other dishes.

Chinese diets

Food and its place in Chinese culture is just as important today as any other period in history and the factors which influenced food habits at home continue to influence them in Britain.

Rice is the staple in China. It is eaten at all meals, either steamed or boiled. In Northern China, wheat, maize and corn are used more than rice. Noodles are another important staple. Fried noodles or chow mein are popular and may be served with other ingredients such as chicken. Soup and noodles can be a substantial meal as the soup usually contains pieces of meat, fish, egg and vegetables.

Vegetables are an important part of the meal and are often quick fried and served with a sweet and sour or soy sauce. Vegetables are always lightly cooked. Chinese meals usually have garlic, fresh ginger and soy sauce as flavourings.

In Britain, traditional food is bought mainly from Chinese grocers. Usually tinned, dried and preserved foods are readily available. Recently, there has been an increase in the number of vegetables available in the large cities.

Certain beliefs influence the food choices of members of the Chinese community. Most elderly Chinese people believe in the concept of 'yin' and 'yang' – the balance of 'hot and cold' or yang and yin energies in the human body. They believe that good health is a state of proper balance between the opposite energies. Illness is the result of an imbalance between the two energies. When the body becomes too 'hot' or too 'cold', diet plays an important part in maintaining the individual's normal healthy balance and in correcting inbalances because different foods have either 'heating', 'cooling' or neutral properties. Old people – whose normal balance is generally cooler than younger people – will be encouraged to eat plenty of hot foods to prevent them from getting too cold. Many Chinese believe that consumption of well boiled soup speeds recovery. The belief of having 'hot' and 'cold' foods for certain conditions is common in the Indian subcontinent as well.

In China, all drinking water must be boiled. Everyone carries a vacuum flask for their daily needs, and public drinking taps also produce boiling water. The offer of cold water may be rejected as impure, and during hospitalisation Chinese people run the risk of dehydration.

Buddha, the founder of Buddhism, advised against gluttony and suggested that moderating the intake of food would help to achieve a long and healthy life.

Afro-Caribbean diets

Food customs observed in the Caribbean Islands are an amalgamation of African, European, Asian, North American and Latin American food practices. Generally, herbs and spices are used substantially in all foods and beverages. Hot sauces, hot peppers and other condiments are also used as flavourings for the dishes.

Patterns of meals in each household are determined by various factors such as economic position, traditional knowledge and experience, availability of foods, convenience of food preparation and, of course, prevailing social norms and values.

Mostly, three main meals are eaten each day. A traditional meal will consist of roots and tubers and starchy fruit like green bananas, bread-fruit, yam and cereals such as rice and wheat flour in different forms. Other components of the meal are meat, fish, poultry, peas, beans and vegetables. These vary in quantity and type, according to economic status.

Caribbean diet consists of the following foods:

- starchy fruit such as yam, sweet potato, cassava, dasheen, green banana and breadfruit etc.;
- cereal grains such as rice, cornmeal, wheat and oats;
- peas, beans (legumes) and nuts;
- dark green/leafy and yellow vegetables which include vegetables such as pumpkin, carrots, kale, callaloo, dasheen and spinach etc.;
- fish and animal foods.

Markets in Afro-Caribbean neighbourhoods sell traditional foods like pulses, coconuts, peanuts, mangoes, cassava, dasheen, breadfruit, okra and green bananas, plaintains and yams.

Problems of elderly ethnic minority groups

The elderly population of minority groups share many of the problems of the indigenous elderly – for example, decreasing mobility, failing health, loneliness, poverty, mental disturbance and ignorance. Traditionally, the elderly from minority groups had a senior position in their family giving them influence over family matters; but this is being put to the test by children born in this country. The system of extended families has started to change in the young British Asians, causing distress and emotional problems to members of the older generation.

Elderly populations from minority groups can suffer from malnutrition in a similar way to the indigenous elderly groups.

Factors leading to poor nutrition in the elderly can be broadly divided into three main groups (see Table 17.1). Malnutrition can be real; for example, a British or Anglicised elderly patient living mainly on a diet of fish and chips or sausage and chips is very likely to suffer from folic acid deficiency. Similarly, vegetarians are prone to develop iron deficiency anaemia because the body absorbs more iron from animal proteins than from vegetable sources. It is important that the appropriate nutritional supplements are provided.

Table 17.1   Factors leading to poor nutrition in the elderly

Social	Loneliness
	Poverty
	Ignorance
	High alcohol intake
	Institutional catering
Psychological	Mental disturbance
	Dementia
	Confusion
	Depression
Physical	Physical disability
	Immobility/being housebound
	Arthritis, especially of hands
	Blindness/partial sight
	Poor dentition
	Decreased sense of taste and smell

It is widely accepted that there are clinical benefits to supplemental feeding of the elderly patient in acute illness. It is not realised sufficiently that nutritional depletion during rehabilitation may be more serious than during the acute illness because the rehabilitation period may extend over weeks or months. Continued suppression of appetite during the rehabilitation period is more likely when patients are offered unfamiliar or unacceptable food (Williams, 1990). Care staff can help patients from different religions by avoiding taboo foods (see Chapter 7). Provision of culturally familiar food in the convalescent period can promote recovery. Asians are one of the largest ethnic minority groups in Britain but, culturally, they are a heterogenous group. In spite of this it is easy to learn the basic differences. The choice of food, whether Indian or English diet, will also depend on the length of settlement in Britain and how eager or successful the patient has been in being assimilated into Western culture. For example, same Kenyan Asians might be more Westernised than those who come from the Asian subcontinent. Before food is offered, the patient should be asked about food taboos otherwise they may be made to feel very guilty and become extremely unhappy. Spitting out food given may be misinterpreted. Such suffering can be prevented.

Effects of medical intervention

Interventions experienced by the ill elderly may include surgery, fasting for tests, and drugs.

Certain drugs may affect nutrition by impairing the appetite, causing nausea and altering the sense of taste. Some elderly people might be using their traditional remedies. These can sometimes be herbal. Most of the elderly from minority groups strongly believe in hot and cold foods. They may include some of their foodstuffs in the diet as medication.

The elderly in residential homes

The quality and quantity of food provided to elderly people within a continuing care hospital or home are obviously important. Cooking procedures, presentation of food and choice are also important considerations. This includes the serving of food by care assistants, nurses and other personnel. They need to be aware that their attitudes may prejudice the acceptance of food. This is even more important when the food is different from that of the carer. Nutritional status and the dietary requirements of institutionalised elderly have attracted considerable attention in recent years (Platt *et al.*, 1985). The question raised was whether elderly people are disadvantaged by nutrient intake below the recommended daily amounts. If that is the case with people who are served meals they are familiar with, it is difficult to imagine what happens to elderly people from a minority group who are served a type of food they have never eaten in their life. The nutritional status of such clients is bound to be lower. This situation may become still worse when the individual concerned is unable to communicate and express his or her views.

Various studies have shown that the ascorbic acid content of foods served in the hospital or institutions is low, mainly because of losses during preparation, processing and distribution of food.

Requirements of the elderly

There is relatively little information on the specific nutritional needs of the elderly. It is assumed that energy requirements fall because of decreased activity. The elderly of all ethnic groups may require a more nutrient dense diet than their younger counterparts and more careful planning of the diet would be necessary. The question has arisen whether the Recommended Dietary Allowances are of any value as the physiological processes, including absorption, differ from the younger age group (Schneider *et al.*, 1986).

Energy and protein requirements are increased, however, in certain conditions such as pressure sores and fever. These conditions tend to depress the appetite which can lead to dramatic weight loss. The extent and duration of such an affect should be monitored. High energy and protein supplements might be required to prevent weight loss.

The DHSS (1979) Survey found the incidence of malnutrition in people aged over 75 years to be 7 per cent, but this figure was doubled for those over 80 years.

Within the next decade, there will be a 45 per cent increase in the numbers of people aged 85 years and over – the frailest section of the elderly population who demand most in terms of health and social services.

What are the guidelines for healthy eating and how relevant are these to the elderly from minority groups? Current nutritional recommendations suggest that, in general, we should do the following.

- Reduce the total fat we eat by a quarter. Our present intake of fat has been linked with heart disease and obesity. If someone is overweight, it is advisable to cut down on fat as it is a concentrated source of calories. Any damage to arteries has long since been done and is not reversible. Fat soluble vitamin A and D are important to all elderly people, especially vitamin D.

- Reduce sugar intake by half. At present, we are having lots of sugary snacks and drinks, especially between meals. Excess of sugar is associated with dental decay, obesity and diabetes. Need to reduce sugar only if overweight or diabetic. Sugary foods may decrease the appetite of other foods as sugar is only empty calories.

- Eat less salt. Most of us eat more salt than we require. Salt keeps blood pressure high and can lead to heart disease. Reduce salt only on medical advice. Some old people suffer from taste changes and reducing salt may make the food less palatable.

- Increase fibre intake by half. Our present low intake has been linked with diabetes, heart disease and cancer. Increasing cereal fibre will improve bowel function and prevent constipation, reducing the need for laxatives and enemas. Having more fibre will benefit everyone. Vegetarian diets are high in fibre and can be encouraged.

How can the professionals and carers help?

Professionals and carers need to recognise the good aspects of traditional diets which are followed by the minority groups, and make sure that undue pressure is not put on elderly people due to ignorance on the part of their carers. This may lead to minority elders undervaluing their traditional diets as some youngsters have started doing.

Regardless of race and creed, reasons for making food choices are remarkably similar. Figure 17.1 summarises the factors which affect eating behaviour.

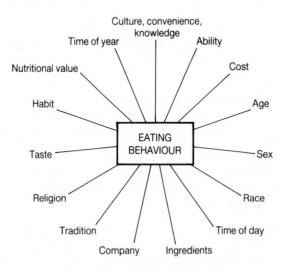

Table 17.1 Factors leading to poor nutrition in the elderly

Practical suggestions

1.   There is a need for in-service training for the carers and professionals dealing with this age group. Certain customs may be associated with meals. For example, hands are always washed before and after the meals; the mouth is rinsed with water after a meal. These are healthy customs and carers should make provisions to enable them to be fulfiled.

2.   When providing special aids to help clients with eating, cutlery plays an important role. It is no use offering a special fork and knife to an Indian or Chinese person who has never used those for eating. If someone is eating with chopsticks, make sure that the food given is in bite size pieces.

3.   Softer diets may be required for residents who have no teeth or ill-fitting dentures and dental advice sought; for those who have problems with chewing, following a stroke; and for people with swallowing problems due to narrowing of the oesophagus.

   Try to use soft foods used by the cultural group. If you need more information, discuss with the relatives or family. Let the clients choose foods they fancy. There may be need to give smaller portions of food, hence little and often feeding may be required.

4.   Liquidised meals should be used as the last resort. By adding water to the food, the nutrients are diluted. Discuss liquidised foods with the dietitian who may suggest ways of improving nutrition. When puréed or liquidised foods are to be served, pay special attention to the presentation.

5.   When advising about the store cupboard for an elderly person living alone, try to include foods which are acceptable culturally.

6.   Diabetes and coronary heart disease are very high among people of the Indian subcontinent. Stroke and hypertension are high among people of Afro-Caribbean origin. If their diets need alteration, consult the dietitian who will then advise according to the traditional foods eaten.

7.   Where budgets for food are tight, advice should be given on how some of the local foods can be included in the meals.

8.   For better uptake of meals in luncheon clubs, day centres or meals-on-wheels, it is better to employ cooks from a similar background. It is probably economical to have central kitchens in a district. These kitchens can then cook Asian vegetarian/ non-vegetarian, Afro-Caribbean and Chinese meals which can then be transported.

9.   Where nutrition education is concerned, it is better to be done by someone who understands the culture very well and can give suggestions of healthy eating in line with current recommendations interpreting that into different cultural foods. It is important to respect the wishes of those who adhere to their known way of life, including dietary constraints. Change should not be imposed nor suggested for the sake of conformity.

10. Be prepared to encourage and support people who are easily discouraged. A little of what they fancy may do them good.

11. Lastly, encourage clients to participate in discussion, even if language is a problem. Positive reinforcement is very important.

Conclusion

Like their younger counterparts, elderly people require food that is palatable, attractively served in pleasant surroundings and at the right temperature. They may be more likely than younger people to choose only food they are familiar with, and to have a preference for 'home style' cooking.

The nutritional intake of elderly people relates closely both to physical and to mental health. It also reflects on their social well-being, but economic, psychosocial and physical factors also play a very important role in nutrition among the aged.

Care of the elderly by family members has been part of the tradition of people from the Indian subcontinent. In Asia, most of the families are extended families. However, this tradition is fast changing on migration. The two reasons for the changes are firstly, small houses; and secondly, the increasing emphasis on individualism as a result of Westernisation. The changing traditional values will have a significant impact on the care of the growing elderly population of the minority groups.

Food habits are an indicator of identity as much as dress, language or religion, ethnic identity and cultural food habits support one another.

It is very clear that members of the first generation, elderly population from a minority group are going to look for traditional foods to recreate themselves in a new country. Our approach towards this group of the community should be practical. It is very difficult to change lifelong eating habits. Carers and professionals need training and awareness courses on the rehabilitation of minority elders.

> For immigrants to change to a traditional British diet, which some claim may play part in our high incidence of coronary artery disease, as well as certain gut diseases, might be to escape from the frying pan into the fire.
>
> BMJ, 1979

References

DEPARTMENT OF HEALTH AND SOCIAL SECURITY (1979). *Nutrition and Health in Old Age*. HMSO, London.

SCHNEIDER, E. L., VINING, E. M., HADLEY, E. C. and FARNHAM, S. A. (1986). Recommended dietary allowances and the health of the elderly. *New England Journal of Medicine*, 314 (34): pp. 157–60.

Further reading and resources

Publications

BENDEN, A. E. (1984). Institutional malnutrition. *British Medical Journal*, 188: pp. 92–3.

CARLSON, E., KIPPS, M. and THOMSON, J. (1984). Influences on the food habits of some ethnic minorities in the United Kingdom. *Human Nutrition: Applied Nutrition*, 38A: pp. 85–98.

EXTON-SMITH, A. N. and CAIRD, F. I. (1980). *Metabolic and Nutritional Disorders in the Elderly*. John Wright, Bristol.

HO, S., DONNAN C., and SHAM, A. (1988). Dietary intake among elderly Chinese in Hong Kong. *Journal of Human Nutrition and Dietetics*, 205–15.

MACLENNAN, W. J., MARTIN, P. and MASON, B. J. (1975). Causes of reduced dietary intake in a long-stay hospital. *Age and Ageing*, 4: pp. 175–80.

SHUKLA, K. (1980). *Diet and Culture. Nursing*, April.

SHUKLA, K., RUCK, N. and FORREST, D. (1980). Feeding practices in the Asian community. *MIMS Magazine*, 15 December: 21–9.

WATSON, R. R. (1985). *Handbook of Nutrition in the Aged*. CRC, Boca Raton.

WILLIAMS, C. M. (1990). Nutritional demands during rehabilitation from acute illness. *Geriatric Medicine*, 20 (6): 33–6.

Training packs

Henley, A. *Asian Foods and Diets.* Available from the National Extension College, 1 Brooklands Avenue, Cambridge, CB2 2HN.

Afro Caribbean Foods and Diets and *Chinese Foods and Diets*. Training packs including slides from Training in Health and Race, 229 Woodhouse Lane, Leeds L52 9LF.

Video

Asian Mother and Baby Campaign. A *Taste of Health – A Video on General Nutrition for Asians*.

18

Ethnic minority elders and the pharmacy

Alison Blenkinsop, Rhona Panton and Indoo Partop

The elderly, that is women aged over 60 and men aged over 65 years, receive a significantly higher number of prescriptions than other groups in the population. In the United Kingdom during the year 1988, elderly patients were prescribed, on average, 17.4 prescription items compared with a national average of 5.6 items (Department of Health, 1988). With this higher number of medicines and their benefits comes a range of potential problems, including drug interactions and adverse reactions or side effects.

Recent research has shown the consultation rate with general medical practitioners to be higher for patients in some ethnic groups (Balara Jan *et al.*, 1989; Gillam *et al.*, 1989). This increased consultation rate is likely to be accompanied by a higher rate of prescribing. Ethnic minority elders are thus potentially likely to receive a high number of prescriptions.

There is great potential for community pharmacists to have a positive influence on the health of their customers. Surveys have shown that 78 per cent of elderly people always use the same pharmacy when they collect their prescriptions (Cartwright and Smith, 1988). There is thus the opportunity to build up a good relationship with the pharmacist and for the pharmacist to be aware of the range of medication being taken.

Elderly people make up a large proportion of pharmacy customers because of the high likelihood that they are receiving prescribed medication. They also seek advice from the pharmacist about minor ailments and their treatment. In particular, purchases of over-the-counter laxatives and painkillers are common. The opportunities for pharmacists to give advice to ethnic minority elders about their medicines and about general health matters are, therefore, considerable.

For ethnic minority elders, there are two major issues: firstly, the problems of medicine-taking in old-age; and, secondly, differences in language and culture, which can significantly influence health (Henley, 1979).

Pharmacy-based research to look at the needs of ethnic minority patients is, to date, limited. Studies to date (Kaur and Dobrzanski, 1988; Partop *et al.*, 1986; Wiggins, 1990) include consideration of an inner city Birmingham health district which has a high proportion of Asian residents and a smaller percentage of Afro-Caribbeans, also a survey of the use of community pharmacies by Asian patients. This chapter considers the findings of existing research in its attempts to identify potential problem areas as well as some possible solutions for pharmacists (Kaur and Dobrzanski, 1988).

Problems of old age in relation to medicine taking

Increasing age brings with it a likelihood of poor eyesight, hearing loss, and the progression of diseases such as arthritis so that dexterity can be greatly reduced. All these problems have implications for pharmacy practice and the giving of advice. Patients with poor eyesight may be unable to read medicine labels, particularly where computer ribbons are badly worn and in need of replacement, thus printing faintly. The additional labels which are attached to medicine bottles often have very small print which may be difficult to read. Some computers offer a facility to print in larger type, and employing this can be helpful. For patients who are blind, or whose eyesight is very poor, standard medicine labels are available as plastic tags with instructions in Braille.

Patients who are hard of hearing may find communication with the pharmacist difficult. Here it is important for the pharmacist to face the patient, to speak slowly and clearly and to offer separate written information about the medicines and how to take them.

The use of child-resistant containers has become widespread in pharmacies in an attempt to limit accidental poisoning in children. Some elderly patients find child-resistant closures very difficult to remove and the Royal Pharmaceutical Society (the pharmacists' professional body) advises pharmacists that, whilst child-resistant closures should normally be used for all medicines, ordinary closures should be used where the patient has difficulty in opening a container. Elderly patients should, therefore, be encouraged to ask the pharmacist for ordinary medicine bottles. Nevertheless, many elderly patients are well able to open child-resistant closures if they are shown how to use them. Where the patient has been unable to open the medicine bottle, there have been situations where medicines bottles have been left open after removing the top or the contents transferred into other containers which may be less suitable. The risk of accidental poisoning is always present and, for those elderly people with young grandchildren, all medicines should be kept out of reach.

Particular problems for ethnic minority elders

Particular concerns are that some patients will not be able to read English and will thus have difficulty in understanding the directions on medicine labels. Where another member of the family is able to read English, a translation will be given, and the same also applies where a pharmacist may give an explanation to an English-speaking member of the family. It should be remembered, though, that these translations will be second-hand (Ahmed *et al.*, 1982) and that the patient may not have the opportunity to ask questions. The study of inner city Birmingham (Partop *et al.*, 1986) found there to be many pharmacies in areas where an Asian language was predominant. In the majority of these pharmacies, either the pharmacist him/herself spoke the language or employed members of staff who did so. There was a small minority of pharmacies where neither the pharmacist nor a member of staff was able to speak the language of many of the pharmacy customers. We think that pharmacists in such areas would be well advised to employ staff members who are able to communicate with customers in their own language.

Prescriptions are issued in over three quarters of patients' consultations with general medical practitioners. Some patients feel that a prescription is a substitute for a fuller discussion of their problems. Such feelings may be intensified where a language barrier exists.

Fasting and medicines

Cultural and religious background can also have an impact on medicine taking. Fasting is a feature of several religions and may be practised by patients including Hindus, Sikhs and Moslems (see Chapter 7). Concern over the constituents of the medicine may be expressed by patients with strong adherence to particular religions and these will also be discussed.

Ramadan (Ramazan) is a month-long period which forms part of the Islamic calendar and is a basic tenet of the Islamic faith. During Ramadan, Moslems are required to abstain from food, tobacco and liquids (including water) between the hours of dawn (an hour or so before sunrise) and sunset. Unsurprisingly, perhaps, concerns have been expressed about patient compliance with prescribed medication during Ramadan, with studies suggesting that as many as three quarters of Moslem patients may not take their medications as prescribed (Aslam and Healey, 1986; Wiggins, 1990).

It is noteworthy that children under the age of 12 are not required to undertake the fast, nor are elderly people (Henley, 1979). Those who are ill need not observe the strict regimen of Ramadan but are required to make a compensatory fast at some other time.

There are about 1.5 million Moslems in the United Kingdom, hence a substantial number of those taking prescribed medication are involved. Some pharmacists and prescribers have suggested that twice daily doses during Ramadan using longer acting or sustained release preparations, or altering the dose regimen, might help to counter the problem (John, 1988; Qazi, 1989). Others have pointed out, however, that there has been no clinical work carried out to investigate the influence of fasting and restricted fluid intake on absorption and serum levels of drugs in this situation (Al-Janabi, 1988). The interpretation of the requirements of Ramadan in relation to drug therapy suggests that only oral preparations are forbidden during the fast period, and topical products, injected drugs and other routes such as the rectal route may be acceptable (Qazi, 1989). Such an interpretation cannot be regarded as definitive however.

Pharmacists need to recognise the practical problems and to discuss possible solutions with both prescribers and patients.

Medicines containing alcohol

As mentioned in Chapter 7, alcohol is forbidden in four religions – Islam, Hinduism, Sikhism and Buddhism. Many oral medicines – as well as topical applications such as lotions, liniments, gels, creams and ointments – contain some form of alcohol. Surgical spirit may contain 75–95 per cent alcohol.

In every religion, some people have liberal views while others have strict traditional beliefs. Patients with liberal views, particularly those educated in Christian countries, may accept alcohol in medicines and local applications. But the traditionalist will not accept alcohol, even as a drug or part of an ointment. It is likely that a devoutly religious person may refuse to accept any form of alcohol in a substance, preferring to die while being loyal to his or her religion rather than live with the guilt of betrayal. Pharmacists can check the alcohol content (if any) of the medicine by referring to the manufacturer, or to the local drug information pharmacist. Discussion with both patient and prescriber may result in the selection of an alternative preparation which does not contain alcohol. The pharmacist must be sensitive to, and recognise the importance of, the patient's concerns about alcohol.

As a last resort, mediation from the appropriate religious leader should be sought.

Gelatin capsules

Gelatin capsules are made from the bones and hide of animals including cows and pigs. A devout Hindu, Sikh, Moslem or Jew (and of course vegetarians and vegans) may not accept a drug in capsule form, including capsules containing antibiotics or with a drug for asthma inhalers. To the unwary, the ethnic minority elders may not have a problem but, to the caring health professional, this should be a matter for concern.

Patients have access to books which tell them which medicines or local applications contain substances which are forbidden in their religions. Where such a problem arises, the pharmacist will need to discuss possible options with the prescriber. It might be possible to give the drug in a different form, for example.

Written information for patients

Patient information leaflets are being used increasingly in pharmacy to supplement information given verbally by the pharmacist. With the advent of original pack dispensing during the 1990s, it is likely that all dispensed medicines will have a patient information leaflet. The difficulties of writing leaflets in such a way that patients are likely both to read and to understand them are well documented. Essentially, the vocabulary used should be simple, sentences should be short, print should be sufficiently large to be easily read, and careful thought should be given to layout and illustrations.

Some drug companies produce leaflets which are written in Asian, Chinese and other languages. Medicines used to treat tuberculosis are an example of where such leaflets are available.

In the past there has been uncertainty about the level of literacy among members of ethnic minorities. A particular myth was that Asian patients who were unable to read English, were unlikely to be able to read at all, and this has been used as an argument against providing written information in Asian languages. Research (Stephens and Fletcher, 1989) has shown that approximately one third of Asian patients are unable to read, a further one third are able to read an Asian language, and the remaining third read either English alone or English and an Asian language. These proportions may vary from area to area, depending on the proportion of first generation immigrants. It is, therefore, worthwhile to consider the production of medicine labels and patient leaflets in Asian languages. Pharmacists can take advice on the appropriate languages from local health promotion units. For example, in the area of Birmingham studied by Partop *et al.* (1986), Urdu and Punjabi were the main languages spoken and read.

Pharmacists who are considering designing patient leaflets for members of ethnic groups should take great care in obtaining translations, since direct translations may not only lose the sense of the information but may actually be offensive. Any such leaflets should be piloted using local community groups of the ethnic minority concerned. As an example of the difficulties which may be encountered, exact translations of medical terms may not exist, so that for Asian patients diabetes has commonly to be referred to as 'sugar problems'. The authors have had some experience in compiling health education leaflets in Urdu and Punjabi as part of a pharmacy-based anti-smoking campaign. The amount of such material available is extremely limited and it would be helpful to have a central point which stocked the full range of materials available. Three quarters of the Asian patients we surveyed thought that the provision of leaflets and labels in Asian languages would be valuable (Kaur & Dobrzanski, 1988). A similar percentage was found in a recent study (Wiggins, 1990).

The language used in both medicine labels and leaflets should be considered carefully by the pharmacist. Unfortunately, pharmaceutical jargon still abounds in instructions on medicine labels, and there is a need for the use of 'plain English' in medicine labelling. Research has shown that members of the public who speak and read English, and where English is the first language, have difficulty in understanding some of the terms used. Classic examples are the use of the word 'instil' (in relation to the use of eye-drops), 'insert' and 'apply'. By the use of larger print, where this is available, and by simplifying the terms used on medicine labels, the pharmacist can do a great deal to improve understanding of written instructions.

Verbal advice from the pharmacist

The giving of advice about the use of prescribed medicines is increasingly recognised as an important part of the pharmacist's role, both in hospital and in the community. Patients and their relatives are increasingly utilising the pharmacy as a source of advice on medicines and general health matters. As we have already said, there will be some situations where the pharmacist is unable to speak the language of ethnic minority clients. Some pharmacy-based research (Partop *et al.*, 1986) has examined the value and acceptability of the pharmacist learning commonly-used dosage instructions in the appropriate language. The drawback of this is that, should the client or patient wish to ask further questions, the pharmacist would not be in a position to understand or answer them. Recognising this, the researchers recommended that efforts should be made to employ bilingual pharmacists in areas where a language barrier existed. Also valuable is the employment of one or more staff members who are able to speak the language concerned. Thus a translation of the appropriate instructions can be given and any questions which the patients wants to ask can be relayed to the pharmacist and then answered. The problems of such translations are well-documented and recognised (Ahmed *et al.* 1982). However, in the circumstances, it is probably difficult to achieve a better system.

Compliance with drug therapy

We know from research that, on average, 50 per cent of the medicines which are prescribed are never taken by the patient. There has been relatively little research which has looked at compliance in ethnic minority patients (with the exception of specific studies on, for example, Ramadan). However, there is a large relevant literature which has looked at patient compliance more generally, and many important points have emerged which are relevant to all patients – particularly those who are elderly. There are various reasons for this, including:

- the patient feels better and stops taking the medicine;
- the patient feels worse and then, rightly or wrongly, attributes this to the medicine;
- the patient's symptoms or condition do not improve, and thus the medicine is discontinued;
- specific directions and instructions are forgotten, hence the medicine is not taken;
- the patient chooses not to take the medicine at all.

Patient understanding and recall have been shown to be of critical importance in relation to compliance. Where multi-drug therapy is involved – and this is often the case with elderly patients – remembering to take each dose, and taking each dose at the appropriate time, can become very difficult. If patients do not understand why they are taking each medicine, it is even more difficult for them to remember and adhere to the dosage instructions. As far as the use of medicines is concerned, some pharmacists have labelled each medicine with its purpose – for example, sleeping tablets, painkillers, etc. since the name of the medicine in itself is unlikely to indicate its use. Where there are language barriers and reading difficulties special efforts are needed to ensure that ethnic minority elders have sufficient information about their medicines.

Various aids are available to improve patient compliance. These include specially designed boxes, with separate compartments for different days of the week or different times of the day, into which the medication is placed. Two sophisticated devices are the *Dosett* and the *Medidos*, comprising portable boxes or trays with separate compartments for different times of day. The box can be filled by the pharmacist, health visitor or a family member who has been trained to do so. more simple devices include egg-box type containers. The 'Beehive' tray simply has four sections which can be labelled 'Breakfast', 'Lunch', 'Supper', 'Bedtime' or other times to suit the individual patient. Pharmacists can, and do, draw up medication charts for patients to help them remember when to take their medicines. Here, the identification of potential language and reading problems is essential.

The problems of compliance are universal but for elderly patients they are particularly acute, and for ethnic minority elders there may be the additional problems of language difficulties. It is very important, therefore, that the elderly patient's ability to understand and remember dosage instructions is assessed so that appropriate additional help can be given where necessary. The importance of taking long term anti-hypertensive treatment or a prolonged course of anti-tuberculosis treatment will need careful explanation and monitoring.

Non-compliance with prescribed therapy, and also over-prescribing, can lead to dramatic amounts of medicines being hoarded in the patient's home. A search of 500 houses resulted in 43 000 unwanted tablets being collected, and in one campaign to collect unwanted medicines 2.25 tons of medicines were found in just one city. Where such campaigns are mounted, information leaflets and posters in the appropriate languages are essential. Posters and other information should be distributed using links with local community groups to ensure they reach the intended audience. The sequence of events between the patients' symptoms or disease, through the healthcare network, to the patients actually taking their treatment has been called 'The Fragile Therapeutic Chain' (Main, 1988) (see Fig. 18.1).

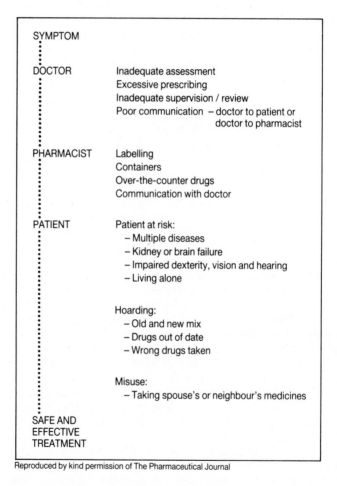

Reproduced by kind permission of The Pharmaceutical Journal

Fig. 18.1 The Fragile Therapeutic Chain (Main 1988)

Adverse reactions in elderly patients

Elderly patients suffer a large number of adverse reactions from the drugs which they take. A survey of geriatric units found that one in every ten admissions was the result of an adverse reaction to drugs. Part of the reason for this large number of adverse reactions is the sheer number of medicines which elderly people take. We have already seen that they take three times more than the average number of drugs. However, there are other reasons for the high incidence and these include changes in the way the body handles drugs, which occur with advancing age, and also changes in the sensitivity of particular parts of the body to drugs.

Absorption and distribution of drugs

The absorption of drugs is little changed with old age. The exception to this is some drugs which are partly broken down in the liver before they get into the bloodstream. These drugs undergo what is called 'first pass metabolism' and in some elderly patients, where the liver is smaller and blood flow within it is reduced, more of the drug can reach the general circulation, i.e., there is increased bio-availability of the drug and stronger effects. It needs to be borne in mind that some ethnic minority groups may vary in their ability to metabolise certain drugs (e.g. isoniazid for tuberculosis) and may also vary in their therapeutic response to drugs (e.g. beta-blockers in Afro-Caribbean hypertensives).

Distribution of a drug in the body depends on the amount of body water (for drugs which are water-soluble) and body fat (for drugs which are lipid-soluble) and on the quantities of special carrier proteins in the blood. All these can be changed in old age. What happens is that water-soluble drugs tend to have a higher blood concentration and thus greater effects (and possibly side effects) in elderly people and fat-soluble drugs have a lower concentration.

The liver and kidneys are the main ways in which the body processes and gets rid of drugs. Basically in old age, the breakdown of drugs in the liver is likely to be reduced, and the filtration rate of the kidneys will also be lower, so that elimination may be decreased and therefore higher blood levels of the drug may result.

Thus the bodies of elderly patients may handle drugs in a quite different way from those of younger patients. For the same dose, the amount of drug which is circulating in the body may be altered, and the effects on drug metabolism are particularly important since they mean that the drug may remain in the body for longer, and at higher levels, than would be the case in a younger person.

Increased sensitivity

The second reason for the higher incidence of adverse reactions in elderly patients is that the 'target organ' may be more sensitive to a particular drug. That means that the drug's effect may be far greater than in a younger patient, and the effect may also last for longer. Examples of this include the more profound effect of nitrazepam and temazepam. Elderly people are particularly prone to 'hang-over' effects from these hypnotic drugs, which can result in confusion, drowsiness and falls, especially if the patient wakes up during the night and moves around. Another common problem in the elderly is that the cardiovascular system responds less quickly to postural changes, so that postural hypotension can be a problem with diuretics and beta blockers, leading to dizziness and falls. It is easy to see that the elderly are therefore more prone to the side effects of drugs, and the prescribing of multiple drug regimes can only add to this problem. Pharmacists and other members of the health care team need to be alert to the possibilities of adverse reactions so that they can be quickly detected. In particular, mental confusion or falls beginning after the start of drug therapy should be investigated.

Patients need to have a greater awareness of the importance of reporting any symptoms to their doctor or pharmacist, and of disclosing the identity of all medicines being taken, Adverse reactions could then be related to medication and appropriate action taken.

Minor ailments and the elderly

Over-the-counter medicines are often purchased and kept in the medicine cupboard by elderly patients. Many of these products are not regarded as drugs or medicines by many members of the public because of their wide availability. The assumption is that anything which can be bought over the counter is harmless and without side-effects. While over-the-counter medicines are undoubtedly safe when taken in the recommended doses, their continued and unsupervised use can lead to problems. For example, Beecham's Powders are sometimes seen as an all round, all purpose medicine, and many people do not know that this product contains aspirin. Antacids which contain aluminium or calcium can lead to constipation, as can painkillers whch contain codeine. Conversely, those antacids which contain only magnesium salts can lead to diarrhoea. Laxatives, too, are widely used and these can lead to dehydration and an imbalance of electrolytes in the body, particularly when the patient is taking diuretics.

Many pharmacies now maintain patient medication records which list the medication history of the patient. Any over-the-counter medicines which are bought should be entered into the patient medication record, firstly to check for the possibility of drug interactions, and secondly so that there is a record of their use. Many elderly people will already be receiving painkillers on prescription, and there is a particular need to be careful with medicines containing paracetamol, where inadvertent duplication may occur if over-the-counter painkillers are taken as well.

Herbal and other folk remedies are widely sold and used, and this is particularly true for some ethnic groups. Transcultural medicine is in itself a speciality, and research has shown that some remedies which are sold, for example, in Asian grocers' shops contain high doses of steroids and other potent drugs. Patients may sometimes be reluctant to disclose that they are taking traditional in addition to Western-style medication but it is very important that they do so because adverse reactions from some of these products can be very dangerous.

What the pharmacist can do to help ethnic minority elders

Pharmacists must recognise the problems in communicating across a language barrier and should take steps to ensure that, in their pharmacy, the language of local ethnic customers is spoken. The predominant languages can be identified through the local health promotion unit.

Verbal information alone is not sufficient and, where possible, pharmacists should try to supplement this by written information in the language of their customers. Such supplementary information could usefully include standard medicine labels with common directions for use and also patient information leaflets.

An awareness of the cultural background of local ethnic groups can help the pharmacist to understand health beliefs and practices, including the use of traditional healers and medicines. For elderly ethnic patients, the pharmacist, or a member of staff, should always check whether child-resistant closures can be opened readily, or whether simple screw-tops are preferred.

Patient medication records should be kept for all elderly customers and should include over-the-counter in addition to prescribed medicines. Closer collaboration between pharmacists and prescribers could help to ensure that appropriate information is given to patients. General practitioners could also help to raise awareness of the pharmacist's role among patients from ethnic minorities.

Closer working between pharmacists and other members of the healthcare team could identify and deal with potential problems. Community pharmacists would welcome closer contact with, for example, district nurses and health visitors in this context.

Finally, research (Partop *et al.*, 1986) has shown that patients from ethnic minorities do not make the best use of pharmacy services. This is partly because of a lack of recognition of the pharmacist as a source of advice. Accessibility to and availability of the pharmacist for answering queries and discussing problems with customers is, therefore, important.

References

AHMED, S., VALENTINE, S. and SHIRE, S. (1982). Translation is at best an echo. *Community Care*, 00: pp. 19–21.

AL-JANABI, T. I. H. (1988). Ramadan (letter). *Pharmaceutical Journal*, 240: pp. 615–6.

ASLAM, M. and HEALY, M. A. (1986). Compliance and drug therapy in fasting Muslim patients. *Journal of Clinical Hospital Pharmacy*, 11: pp. 321–5.

BALARAJAN, R., YUEN, P. and SONI RALEIGH, V. (1989). Ethnic differences in general practitioner consultations. *British Medical Journal*, 299: pp. 958–60.

CARTWRIGHT, A. and SMITH, C. (1988). *Elderly Patients, their Medicines and Their Doctors*. Routledge and Kegan Paul, London.

DEPARTMENT OF HEALTH (1988). *Prescription Statistics*. HMSO, London.

GILLAM, S. J., JARMAN, B., WHITE, P. and LAW, R. (1989). Ethnic differences in consultation rates in urban general practice. *British Medical Journal*, 299: pp. 953–7.

HENLEY, A. (1979). *Asian Patients in Hospital and at Home*. Kings Fund, London.

JOHN, D. N. (1988). Ramadan (letter). *Pharmaceutical Journal*, 240: p. 552.

KAUR, M. and DOBRZANSKI, S. (1988). Pharmacy counselling for patients of Indian Pakistan origin. *British Journal of Pharmacy Practice*, 10: pp. 345–50.

MAIN, A. (1988). Elderly patients and their drugs. *Pharmaceutical Journal*, 240: p. 539.

PARTOP, I., MORLEY, A. and PANTON, R. S. (1986). A survey of patients from ethnic minorities: do they use pharmacy services effectively? *Pharmaceutical Journal*, 237: pp. 724–5.

QAZI, T. U. (1989). Ramadan (letter). *Pharmaceutical Journal*, 242: p. 671.

STEPHENS, K. A. and FLETCHER, R. F. (1989). Communicating with Asian patients. *British Medical Journal*, 299: pp. 905–6.

WIGGINS, H. (1990). Meeting the needs of ethnic minority patients. *British Journal of Pharmacy Practice*, 12: pp. 170–7.

19

Social work with minority ethnic elders

Ruth Prime

Social work with ethnic minority elders cannot be divorced from social work with elderly people in general, since the way in which the needs of the elderly are met, in part, determines the way in which the needs of black and ethnic minority elders will be met.

It is important to note that while many of the needs of black and ethnic minority elders are similar to those of elderly people as a whole, the needs of black and ethnic minority elders are compounded by special features. Common needs, particularly for the elderly in inner cities, are poor housing, low incomes, social isolation, problems of adjustment to increasing age, poor health and impaired mobility; however, where the black and ethnic minority elders are concerned, there are the special features of growing old in a foreign country, loss of role and status in the family, problems of cultural adjustments and racism all of which give rise to feelings of isolation and rejection, and which in turn often lead to depression. These points are well made by Alison Norman (1986), and Kenneth Blackmore (1983). The 1989 White Paper, *Caring for People*, recognises that 'people from different cultural backgrounds may have particular care needs and problems'.

Social work is here used in the broad sense to cover the range of services delivered by local authority and hospital social services departments and the voluntary sector through a process which includes assessment of need and the meeting of need through information giving, counselling, advocacy and the provision of resources.

While we are here concerned with service delivery there are certain key issues which must be addressed by all agencies in order to provide the framework within which field workers can carry out their duties.

The key issues – policy, staffing and training are interrelated. Though each provides scope for wide ranging discussion, they will be dealt with briefly in this chapter.

Policy

Every agency concerned with social work should have a statement of policy and a strategy for implementing that policy or intention. Further, there must be a system for monitoring and reviewing in order to give the strategy viability and credibility.

Sadly, in many local authorities where policy statements for the elderly exist, black and ethnic minority elders are included or tacked on as an afterthought. Such an approach guarantees that black and ethnic minority elders will not be treated as part of the community. In effect, while there is much rhetoric about multi-racial and multicultural communities, policy and planning centres around the indigenous population. It is imperative that policy makers and planners address this issue in consultation with informed members of the black and ethnic minority communities in order to provide the necessary resources and conditions in which fieldworkers can operate.

Allied to policy on the elderly will be the implementation of an Equal Opportunity Policy (EOP) which should include guidelines for recruitment, interviewing/ selection, ethnic recording, staff opportunities and the composition of interviewing panels. Very often an EOP amounts to little more than a statement which is included in advertisements and is no more than a paper exercise.

Staffing

If an effective EOP is in place, the probability of a workforce which reflects a multicultural community will increase. A representative workforce is likely to enhance the quality of service delivery and its sensitivity to the range of community expectations. However, the creation of a multicultural workforce does not in itself guarantee that all sections of the community will receive a service or that the service will be delivered with cultural sensitivity free from racism. The department's strategy and the effective and appropriate use of staff will be the determining factors.

Training

Training of staff is fundamental to the implementation of EOP and of anti-racist strategies. Anti-racist training should assist workers in the understanding of personal and institutionalised racism and in recognising how racist conditioning may affect their feelings and attitudes. If staff lack this understanding, they are unlikely to respond to the anti-racist strategies which are designed, and without this understanding it would be impossible to move on to developing anti-racist strategies for effective service delivery and for dealing with racism in the workplace.

It must be stressed that training for work in a multicultural society should be an underlying theme of all social work training. If preparation for work in a multicultural society is to be treated seriously it cannot be achieved by devoting a few days to the issue of race; it should be an integral unit of all aspects of social services and health and voluntary organisations' training courses, and should be a revised and refined as appropriate.

With the key issues addressed, the foundation will be laid for the field workers to undertake the tasks of identification of need, assessment and service delivery.

Identification of need

Effective service delivery is dependent on the proper Identification and Assessment of Need. In many social services and health authorities, the needs of black and minority ethnic elders in the community are not known. It is often then assumed that because black and ethnic minority elders do not approach social services departments, either they do not exist or they are looked after by relatives. The prevailing myth is 'they look after their own'.

The truth is that while black and ethnic minority communities would like to look after their own, housing and employment often separate families, so many black and minority ethnic elders live alone. Where relatives do the caring they experience the same stress as the indigenous population. This myth must be dispelled if the elders and their carers are to be helped appropriately.

Further, many black and ethnic minority elders do not know what social services can offer. Services need to be publicised through the ethnic press, media programmes, in relevant languages and in language free of jargon. Workers need to reach out to the community through groups, churches or other places of worship and clubs. In short, the identification of need is best done by communicating with and listening to black and minority ethnic communities. The 1989 White Paper states 'Minority communities may have different concepts of community care and it is important that service providers are sensitive to these variations. Good community care will take account of the circumstances of minority communities and will be planned in consultation with them'.

Population breakdown figures, though crude, can serve as a rough guide to the numbers and location of ethnic minority elders in the community. Every local authority should be able to produce figures by wards through its Policy and Planning Department, which will enable workers to embark on specific projects in local communities.

Race Relations advisors have been effective at promoting change and addressing the issue of race and service delivery. The disadvantage is that the community may see the post as a token, especially if established for a limited time. Providers may be concerned at the possibility of raised expectations within limited resources, and the tact of the individual is crucial.

Results of such endeavours take time, and starting small with visible effect will gain support. A project undertaken by Haringay Health Authority was targetted on ethnic minority elders in the district, and enabled identification of the group, its health and social needs, collected views on service delivery and unmet need, and facilitated a forum jointly to review and plan services. The success was dependent on commitment from managers and continuing enthusiasm from all (Kalsi and Constantinides, 1989).

Having gained some idea of the size of the black and ethnic minority population and, through dialogue, some general idea of how they wish their needs to be met, structures should then be constructed to ensure that such needs are met appropriately and sensitively. This is the point at which imagination, flexibility, innovation and a dismantling of conditioned attitudes come into play.

Black and minority ethnic elders, like the indigenous population, should be guaranteed a minimum service. The quality of service begins at reception – the first contact with the agency. Staff should be deployed in such a manner that non-English speaking people seeking help should be able to communicate in their own language. There are various methods of ensuring that staff who can speak the appropriate languages are readily available. Some local authorities employ Asian receptionists who can speak English plus a number of Asian languages. Others ensure that a range of staff who have command of different languages are available at specific times and can see people by appointment.

Assessment of need

Effective initial and ongoing assessment is fundamental to an appropriate delivery service. Assessments should therefore be comprehensive and should focus on enhancing the independence of the client. One must observe the underlying principle of social care: planning for the individual as a whole taking account of his or her total environment and working with informal carers (relatives, friends, neighbours) and formal carers (doctors, community nurses, geriatric health visitors, social services staff) to meet the needs of the individual in a way that acknowledges that individual's independence and preserves his or her dignity. Support is given to this approach by the following statement in the 1989 White Paper:

> The objective of assessment is to determine the best available way to help the individual. Assessment should focus positively on what the individual can and cannot do and could be expected to achieve taking account of his or her personal and social relationships.

An assessment begins at the point of referral. Information given or requested from the referrer should be of a nature which assists in the assessment process. If, for example, a general practitioner is referring a severely handicapped elderly person for a home help, relevant information will determine who is the more appropriate person to make an assessment, an occupational therapist or a home care organiser.

Amazingly, this very important area of work is left largely to chance in most agencies. In this chapter, therefore, it seems appropriate to look at assessment in some depth. An assessment is carried out to determine whether there are factors, the absence or presence of which may have caused problems or had adverse effects on the quality of life. Having identified these factors an evaluation is made, conclusions are drawn and decisions arrived at. There are roughly five stages of an assessment:

- gathering of information;
- evaluating the information;
- drawing conclusions;
- deciding on the action to be taken;
- monitoring and reviewing.

Gathering of information

The gathering of information is an essential precondition to effective assessment of the elderly; it is acquired by all workers concerned with the care of the elderly through in-house training. The important point is that workers understand the purpose and relevance of the information they are seeking, can share it with client, carer, and each other, avoid duplication and record it concisely and accurately.

The gathering of information should embrace the following elements.

1. Health factors   Both physical and mental health must be assessed. Simplistic phrases such as 'chronic bronchitis' or 'confused' are totally inadequate. What is needed is a precise statement of the way in which these disorders impact on the functioning of the individual. Chronic bronchitis for one person could mean not being able to walk more than a few steps without becoming extremely short of breath, while for another it might mean having to avoid hills but being quite capable of getting around on the flat. Obviously the needs of these two people would be different. Similarly, 'confusion' can range from brief periods of forgetfulness to total disorientation, and the cause can vary.

2. Independence It is more helpful to determine what the client can do and move on to what he or she needs help with or is unable to do. The difference in approach is important because too great an emphasis on disability fosters dependence which is not in the best interest of the client.

3. Physical environment People function within their environment. The environment may be conducive in some respects, inconducive in others. It is essential therefore to take a broad view of the environment.

4. Past history Past experiences often have a bearing on the way people react to the present. It is useful therefore to get some idea of the background of elderly individuals whenever possible. For black and ethnic minority elders it also helps in understanding the adjustments which have to be made.

5. Emotional and psychological needs Loss, life crisis, racism, all result in emotional and psychological stress which is often ignored.

6. Communication How people communicate must be seen as a crucial factor in the assessment process. If assumptions are made about what is being communicated, serious misunderstandings, with negative outcomes, can arise. Attention must therefore be given to verbal communication with elders whose first language is not English, to those who express themselves colloquially, to non-verbal communication, and to those whose speech and hearing are impaired.

7. Issues of race which result in differential access to resources and decision making power, disadvantage in employment, racial harassment and hostility, must not be confused with issues of culture. Consideration must be given to the way racism impacts on the life of the individual.

8. Issues of culture which relate to customs, lifestyles, music, food and dance, amongst other aspects, must be understood and respected.

9. Hobbies and interests Knowing what people enjoy doing creates a basis for providing the appropriate pastime activities.

10. Formal networks It is always useful and helpful to know which other caring agencies are involved: health services, doctors (general practitioners or hospital), community nurses, health visitors, physiotherapists, voluntary organisations.

11. Informal networks Friends, relatives, neighbours, the church or other religious bodies, all play a part in caring and preventing or reducing isolation.

12. Carers   Those who carry the main burden of caring should be consulted, and their perceptions and wishes respected. Recognition of their role and acknowledgement that their needs and abilities must be assessed are crucial aspects of the process.

13. Clients themselves   The client's perception and wishes must be respected. Clients must be party to decision making.

Evaluating the information

Each facet of the information gathered interlocks to form a comprehensive picture. Bits of information must not be used in isolation. Too often during the course of an interview, workers begin making decisions based on isolated remarks and determined by availability of resources. This tendency can best be illustrated by the case of the elderly Afro-Caribbean man who, during the course of an interview, mentioned that he was no longer going out to do his shopping. He was immediately offered meals on wheels which he accepted but rarely ate. The reason for not going out to do his shopping was fear. Recent incidents of racial harassment in the neighbourhood had filled him with such fear that he rarely went out. The symptom was treated inappropriately because the cause was not diagnosed. Making sense of the whole is the key to this vital stage of the assessment process which at times may require the involvement of the line manager.

Drawing conclusions

Having formed a comprehensive picture, conclusions are drawn about the way in which the needs of the individual and carer can best be met. Further assessments involving another discipline, joint assessment or multi-disciplinary assessment may be necessary. The tendency to involve too many people in the assessment process must, however, be guarded against.

Deciding on action to be taken

Action can range from assurance, information giving, advice, advocacy, provision of a single service or services, to a care planning meeting of all relevant people involved or likely to be involved coming together to share information, discuss needs and decide on the most appropriate way of meeting these needs. A 'package of care' should then be drawn up. A care planning meeting may involve workers from social services (home helps, day care staff, social workers, occupational therapists); health (general practitioners, community and psychiatric nurses, physiotherapists, geriatricians, psychogeriatricians); voluntary organisations; housing. This is not an exhaustive list of the organisations nor is it a prescription for involving all these people in every care planning meeting. People should be invited if relevant. The appropriate black and minority ethnic representatives should always be present and genuine effort should be made to ensure that the individual and carer are present.
   The 1989 White Paper states:

> Assessments should take account of the wishes of the individual and his or her carer, and of the carer's ability to provide care and where possible should include their active participation. Effort should be made to offer flexible services which enable individuals and carers to make choices.

Some thought needs to be given to the term 'packages of care'. This term has become very popular since the Griffiths Report (1988) but what exactly does it mean? Prime (1984) describes a package of care as a care plan which must be designed to meet the needs of the individual in the most appropriate and effective manner with the minimum of confusion and intrusion.

A written statement should then be drawn up, stating clearly the role of each person involved, identifying the tasks and the person responsible for the carrying out of each task, specifying time limits, setting a timespan within which each goal should be achieved, stating whether they have been achieved, back-up systems, lines of reporting, support to workers and a named key worker to monitor the package. Finally a review date is set.

Monitoring and reviewing

Assessment may either be brief or continuous. Close monitoring and reviewing are essential so that plans can be adapted to meet changing situations.

Service delivery

If assessments are holistic and needs-led, there is a high probability that the service delivered will be sensitive and appropriate to the needs of black and minority ethnic elders and their carers. Of the range of services available to elders, four will be discussed in order to assist in the achievement of appropriate service delivery. The four services are counselling, day care, residential care and domiciliary services.

Counselling

The need for counselling of elders is often ignored. There is an emphasis on practical help which, though necessary, is not always sufficient. Like everyone else there are times when elders need counselling. Many elders suffer loss in various areas of their lives – loss of income, health, relatives, friends, loved ones, status, independence and dignity. Such losses can lead to depression. For black and ethnic minority elders there are the additional losses: loss of role and status within the family and loss of the dream of returning home.

Loss of role and status within the family can cause great distress to black and minority ethnic elders who, in their countries of origin, would have been respected because of their age and wisdom. In this country because housing and employment often lead to the break up of the family, the role of the head of the family is weakened. Second generations, by absorbing some of the Western culture, have views and ideas which do not always accord with those of their parents so that while children love and respect parents, differences of perception can lead to the rejection of some of the values of the older generation. Black and minority ethnic elders who find themselves displaced as the head of the household and their values rejected can, as a result, experience great distress.

The unfulfilled dream of returning home dawns suddenly and with devastating effect. Throughout their working lives many black elders are sustained by their dream, and suddenly they realise that fulfillment is financially impossible. They have therefore to face the prospect of growing old in a foreign land, a prospect which entails considerable cultural adjustment, at times coming up against racism when they are their most vulnerable. It takes only a little imagination to appreciate the grief and pain which can ensue.

While not advocating that every black and minority ethnic elder will have this experience it is essential that all those who work with these elders are aware that these distressing elements must be taken into account and counselling made available when necessary.

Day care

One of the stated purposes of day care is the relief of isolation. Black and ethnic minority elders can be even more isolated in a day care centre if the 'service for all' attitude prevails. Prime (1987) found that black ethnic minority elders in day care and residential establishments were not provided with appropriate food and leisure activities and that they were subjected to varying degrees of racist abuse from white elders. Staff, unable to deal with the situation, ignored it on the grounds that one cannot change the attitudes of the elderly. The black elders were then left with the choice of not attending day centres or putting up with the abuse. Either way they were left to deal with the pain and humiliation.

All staff have a responsibility to deal with racism in the workplace and managers must ensure that staff are trained and assisted to discharge this responsibility.

Residential care

The purpose of residential care is to provide an alternative home for those who are no longer able to cope in their own home. The Wagner Report (1987) states:

> Living in residential care should be a positive experience ensuring a better quality of life than the residents could enjoy in any other setting.

The Longmans dictionary defines 'home' as 'a congenial environment'.

Where black and minority ethnic elders are concerned, residential care in practice is far removed from the theory. The reality is that black and minority ethnic elders often find residential care a hostile environment that is both physically and emotionally distressing. As discussed above, black and minority ethnic elders in residential care face isolation, deprivation of familiar foods and leisure activities and racist abuse. By no stretch of the imagination can such an environment be described as congenial or the experience positive.

A survey of Afro-Caribbean elders in South London (Boyce, 1990) confirmed the feelings of isolation, and in residential care diet, physical care, recreation and leisure, religion, language and companionship were emphasised. There was a mixed response to provision solely for one group, but a feeling that, although the black community shared some responsibility for its elders, the state provision to which they had contributed should also provide support. The recommendation of the study was that a Day/Residential Resource Centre be set up for black elders to provide a central point for information, training, advocacy and identity, to facilitate independence, but that residential care should be supported when it was necessary.

A number of positive steps need to be taken by social services and housing managers if a sensitive service is to be provided. All workers also have a role to play by constantly drawing attention to the type of service that is needed, but an awareness of the needs of black and minority ethnic elders must precede prescription of services.

Ideally, a number of alternatives to residential care should be found. Wagner (1987) said that 'people who move into residential accommodation should do so by positive choice'. If there are no alternatives, there is no choice. Among the alternatives are: appropriate domiciliary services tailored to meet the needs of the individual; greater support for carers; adult care with matching black and ethnic minority carers to elders; small group homes and sheltered housing for specific ethnic groups.

In spite of these alternatives, a small number of black and ethnic minority elders may eventually need residential care, thus urgent thought must be given to the method of provision. In some instances it might be appropriate to devise systems within existing establishments; in others separate provision would be warranted. Where existing establishments are used it would be helpful to revise admission procedures to ensure that residents and relatives are appropriately received. First impressions must be positive. A member of staff of the same ethnic origin being on duty at the time of a visit or admission could make a considerable difference. Pictures on the walls reflecting the multicultural composition of the home, familiar and personal items in one's room, appropriate food and leisure activities all contribute to a congenial atmosphere. Imagination and commonsense are powerful assets. Just imagine a group of indigenous elderly doing reminiscence exercises. They may talk about the war, tea dances, sing familiar songs and all together recall incidents relevant to this country. An Afro-Caribbean or Asian elder would be isolated in such a group. Finally, like day care staff, residential care staff must be trained to deal with racism in the workplace.

Domiciliary services

Of the services delivered to the elderly in their own home the two most popular and familiar are the home care service and meals on wheels.

Home care service In all social services departments, the vast majority of elderly people receiving a service do so through the home care service. For many elderly people the home care service is vital to the quality of their life, yet relatively few black and ethnic minority elders use the service. It is very easy to assume that black elders neither want nor need the service. The truth is either that they are unaware of the service, or that the service offered is not appropriate to their specific language, cultural or religious needs. Some home helps are often the only, or one of the few, links between the elderly and the outside world; it would therefore make an enormous difference to the quality of their life if black and ethnic minority elders can be supported by home helps with whom they could communicate with ease and who were very likely to understand their cultural and religious needs. Innovative work has been undertaken on this subject with the production of a video (Age Concern, 1989) for training purposes.

The wisdom of recruiting home helps from different cultures has been recognised for several years but it is only within recent times that some social services departments have seriously begun recruitment drives. Another point worth considering is that, since the number of elderly people referred to the home care service far outweighs the number referred through the social work service, there is a strong case for greater liaison between the two services to ensure that the needs of the elderly are identified and met appropriately.

Meals on wheel   Whenever the provision of services for black and ethnic minority elders is discussed, 'meals on wheels' crops up. Many people are of the view that it is the only service required, yet few social services departments have managed to provide a service. Some of the reasons put forward are lack of financial resources and the difficulty of providing the service without knowing demand. Neither is a good enough reason. Budgets are to meet community needs and resources should be allocated to meet the needs of all sections of the community. The 'demand-and-supply' argument could go on forever without resolution so action must be taken. Discussion with the community can identify even a small number of people who need the service and imaginative steps can be taken to meet the need. It might be that catering could be done by a member of the community while the demand is small and contingency plans made for meeting increasing demands. Social service workers at all levels must free themselves of the rigidity with which they deliver services.

Working with other agencies

Social services departments do not possess all the skills and resources to meet all the needs of the elderly. It is therefore incumbent on each social services department to set up structures which enable them to work in an integrated and co-ordinated way with health, housing and the voluntary sector (particularly the black voluntary sector). There must also be a willingness on the part of these agencies to work together for the benefit of the clients and to address all the issues previously outlined.

Many social services have structures for liaising with other agencies at formal (Joint Consultative Committees), and informal (working parties, planning groups) levels; few however have representatives from black and ethnic minority communities who are knowledgeable about the needs of the elderly. Even in social service departments where good structures for families and children exist, the fact that they can be used as models for the elderly seem to go unnoticed.

Health Service

The Health Service plays a major role in the care of the elderly. In many instances black and ethnic minority elders who never approach social services are in contact with the Health Service. Health workers must therefore be sufficiently aware of, and sensitive to, the needs of black and ethnic minority elders to be able to offer appropriate help and refer to social services.

Housing

Most housing departments have a forum with social services to discuss special housing needs which include the needs of the elderly. Few, however, give particular attention to the needs of black elders, who continue to live in some of the poorest housing. Health, social services and housing provide accommodation in some form for the elderly. Good liaison between these agencies and the voluntary sector could lead to a better use of existing resources and alternative ways of meeting housing needs.

Voluntary sector

At present, services for black and ethnic minority elders are in the main provided by small black voluntary organisations. Many of these small organisations provide services in poor premises with inadequate amenities while in some instances the facilities provided by social services are underused.

With limited funding, these voluntary organisations are expected to provide services at a much lower cost than social services and without the guidance and support necessary, particularly in the early stages when they are struggling to establish themselves.

The role of the black voluntary sector as service providers has never been clarified by social services. They have always been seen as a cheap alternative or main providers helped by social services. Now more than ever in the light of the 1989 White Paper, social services must think carefully of the role of the black voluntary sector.

One of the key objectives of the White Paper is:

> . . . to promote the development of a flourishing independent sector alongside good quality public services. The government has endorsed Sir Roy Griffith's recommendation that social services should be 'enabling' agencies. It will be their responsibility to make maximum possible use of the private and voluntary providers and so increase the available options and wider consumer choice.

Many black and ethnic minority elders have a limited choice – the black voluntary sector. Unlike the white indigenous elderly who are provided for from mainstream funding, they are dependent on limited funding from grant aid. This is a denial of the fact that they are part of the community. If social services fail to recognise the need to plan services for black and ethnic minority elders or to accept their responsibility to increase the available options and wider consumer choice, it is very likely that they will take the relevant steps to ensure that black voluntary organisations are enabled to provide an effective service. This would be very unfortunate as black voluntary organisations do not have the same technical skills to fight for recognition and resources as the large conventional organisations. Instead of flourishing the black voluntary sector will die, and black and ethnic minority elders will be dealt a deadly blow.

Conclusion

In this chapter the idea has not been to attempt to cover every aspect of social work with black and ethnic minority elders, but to raise awareness of all those concerned with the care of the elderly, of the issues which underpin good practice.

The key issues of policy, training, and staffing, which provide the framework for service delivery are mainly the concern of management but each individual must take responsibility for dealing with personal racism and for carrying out the policies of the department where they exist or pressing for policies where they do not exist.

If good practice is observed and a more comprehensive and co-ordinated approach is taken, all members of the community will benefit and better use will be made of resources. For black and minority ethnic elders however, appropriate service delivery will only be guaranteed if conditioned attitudes are dismantled and a more flexible, imaginative and innovative approach is taken.

In conclusion it must always be remembered, firstly that communities are dynamic entities which change, as do their needs. It follows then that continuous monitoring and updating of knowledge of the needs of the community are essential features of an effective supportive programme.

Secondly, the tendency to see ageing as a totally negative experience with the elderly being a burden to society must not be encouraged. Among the black and ethnic minority elders there is a wealth of knowledge, skills, ideas and energy which lie unharnessed in the community, because of negative stereotyping.

Finally, if every worker in health, social services, housing and the voluntary sector accepts some responsibility and takes up the challenge, positive change will certainly be brought about.

References

AGE CONCERN (1989). *According to Need* (Video). Age Concern, Mitcham.

BLACKMORE, K. (1983). Their needs are different. *Community Care*, 449: pp. 12–13.

BOYCE, W. (1990). Developing a resource centre for black Afro-Caribbean elders. *Baseline (Journal of the British Association for Service to the Elderly)*, 44: pp. 2–19.

'GRIFFITHS REPORT' (1989). *Community Care – Agenda for Action*. HMSO, London.

KALSI, N. and CONSTANTINIDES, P. (1989). *Working Towards Equality in Health Care: The Haringay Experience*. Kings Fund, London.

NORMAN, A. (1986). *Triple Jeopardy: Growing Old in a Second Homeland*. Centre for Policy on Ageing, London.

PRIME, R. (1984). No longer a second class service. *Community Care*, 536: pp. 25–29.

PRIME, R. (1987). *Developing Services for Black and Minority Ethnic Elders in London: Overview and Action Plan*. Social Services Inspectorate, Department of Health, London.

'WAGNER REPORT' (1987). *A Positive Choice: Residential Care – Report of Independent Review*. HMSO, London.

WHITE PAPER (1989) *Caring for People – Community Care in the Next Decade and Beyond*. HMSO, London.

Section III The Way Forward: Planning Health and Social Services with Ethnic Minority Elders in Mind

20

The way forward: education

Liz Stewart

George Kelly, an eminent psychologist came to the conclusion that, in order to be of real use, helpers must 'put on a clients shoes and walk in their world with them'.

One of the dangers of reading a textbook crammed with information is that we then believe ourselves fully to be informed and ready to take on the world with another's shoes quite comfortably in place. However this is not always the case, particularly where cultural information is concerned. If I say, 'the British eat fish and chips', you would doubtless agree that this is a correct assumption. The reality is that 25 per cent of the population do so on a regular basis, therefore what is seen as a British tradition is in fact untrue for 75 per cent of the people. Therefore to have a healthy eating publicity campaign aimed at reducing the consumption of just fish and chips, would prove to be somewhat wide of the mark. This may lead us to question other cultural assumptions such as that Roman Catholics eat fish on Fridays, or all female Sikhs are known by the name Kaur.

Any judgements we may make in regard to a client needs to be checked out. A good way to check out information verbally, either directly with a client or relative or through an interpreter is to say, 'my understanding of your religion/culture/ nationality leads me to believe that you may . . . am I correct?' This approach indicates that you have a level of expertise but that you will rely on them for verification, not on your own assumptions.

It may seem then that this chapter is about to deny much that has already been written. Not so; what is important is to differentiate between facts and assumptions, particularly assumptions about the needs of others. There is of course a dichotomy here: professional people who are supposed to be expert in their field are perceived to have the wisdom that they then in turn impart to others. But then again, to be aware of one's deficiencies is in itself a skill.

Assumptions and stereotypes are interesting. The origin of the word 'stereotype' comes from 'printing plates which take an image in cast and reproduce it with monotonous regularity. The image is fixed in all details'. The word is used to describe fixed images which individuals, consciously or subconsciously, hold in their minds about different groups of people. The effect is that characteristics are attributed to an individual based on a generalisation (which is usually inaccurate) about a group. What happens when we become acquainted with someone from a commonly stereotyped group? Usually one of three things happen to one's stereotype:

- it vanishes and is replaced by the acceptance of diversity within that group;
- it remains in place and 'exceptions' are allowed;
- the picture is amended and takes on the characteristics of the known person.

You might like to play this game. With each of the following invented people, based on the information given, what do you think you might imagine these people might look like, what is their religion, their ethnicity, their lifestyle, what do they eat, what do they wear?

- Mrs Ethel Green, 80, old-aged pensioner, retirement home, Brighton.
- Mr Isaiah Johnson, 72, old-aged pensioner, terraced home, Brixton.
- Reverend John Freeman, 61, vicar, detached home, Cumbria.
- Mr Mohammed Patel, 29, shopkeeper, maisonette, Southall.
- Ms Ann Bishop, 25, social worker, studio flat, Putney.
- Mrs Indira Desai, 75, housewife, semi-detached home, Manchester.
- Mr Michael Cohen, 53, solicitor, Golders Green.

The most interesting thing to note, however, is not what your 'picture' looked like, but more probably the ease and speed of its development. This exercise was 'easy' because of the number of 'stereotype' clues given. Try it again omitting, say, the occupations, or the locations – does that change your picture? Now, if possible, compare your picture with that of a colleague. How similar or dissimilar are they. The more minimal the information given the more diverse the pictures will become.

Why do we have them? Our brains usually try to make sense of new information as quickly as possible so that we feel safe. Stereotypes provide a framework which accelerates this process because they provide a quick and easy method of assimilating information which creates the illusion of safety.

If I walk into a room containing a number of people, logic tells us that all that could safely be assumed about me is my gender, and within five years or so, my age. Yet consciously or subconsciously assumptions about ethnicity, education, social class, political affiliations, possible areas of employment and marital status will have been deduced from a variety of factors such as how I enter the room, eye contact with those in the room, hairstyle, make up and how I am dressed, the latter being a major message giver. Not that this is in any way wrong – it is only human nature after all – the problems arise only when we make decisions about how we will behave, based on these indeterminate variables.

If we make a 'decision' about someone we are quite naturally keen to prove that we have been correct in our assumptions, and in that aim the odds are weighted that this will be a self fulfilling prophecy as we seek evidence to prove that we were right.

Carl Rogers (1942) coined the phrase 'positive unconditional regard' as being an essential element of a helper/client relationship, but it can be helpful in all sorts of both private and professional situations. This places an emphasis on the importance of an empathic relationship rather than one based on sympathy. The latter of course has its place but an emphatic understanding of others is more dynamic, indicating a willingness to help within the perspective or sphere of another, rather than from personal expectation based on a helper's own values. According to one explanation, there is a person in a ditch, the sympathetic helper jumps into the ditch with him, the empathic helper takes the hand of the person in the ditch and pulls him out. This at first looks and sounds realistic. However the truly empathic helper would first want to know why the person was in the ditch in the first place and how he felt about being in the ditch, before making any assumptions about whether the ditch was a bad place to be.

A good way to demonstrate empathy with a client is to paraphrase or précis in your own words the information he or she is giving you. This indicates that you have been listening and helps your client to trust you. Moreover, this skill is particularly useful to check mutual comprehension when there is a need to collect a lot of detailed information.

To any communication or interaction with others, we bring ourselves and our own values; in order to understand and to celebrate the values of others we need first to look at our own.

What are personal values? How do they differ from beliefs or attitudes? How do we get them?

Established wisdom suggests that the difference between a value and a belief or attitude is that a value is something we will get up and physically do something about. The model shown in Fig. 20.1 may be helpful. Looking at ourselves this way suggests that we hold a myriad of beliefs, on every possible subject, many of which are likely to be unspoken. A strongly held belief is likely to become an attitude about which we may be more verbal. A strongly held attitude is likely to become a value and the sum of our values therefore form our personality. For example, one might feel that the poll tax is a supremely unfair imposition on the community, and would probably sign a petition to that effect. Would one, however, march, risk getting caught up in a violent situation and mistakenly arrested? On balance, no, probably not. Many peoples' personal values are concerned with the need for love, friendship, natural justice and efficient domestic appliances; and they will be quite active in the pursuit and maintenance of these.

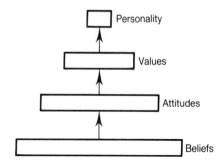

Fig. 20.1   Values, attitudes and beliefs

Individually, our early values will be ones handed down to us from our parents and teachers and these are likely to reflect our culture, socio-economic grouping, religion and nationality. As we get older some of our values are challenged, as we receive more external stimuli and our opinions are modified by peer groups, the media, the status quo, the education system and the experience of discrimination in one form or another.

On the basis that everyone in the world has had a different experience of life, a different set of values and an individual expectation of life, probably the most ineffectual statement one human being can offer another is 'If I were you', or indeed any assumption that what we want for ourselves would meet the needs of another.

A major area for consideration is how much 'authority figures' are an issue, and this is quite likely to be a particular concern for black and ethnic minority elderly people. Let us imagine how our own behaviour may alter, say, when seeing a hospital consultant, being stopped by the police or dealing with the Inland Revenue. How much does our behaviour change? How deferential might we become? How grateful might we be for help? How much do deference and gratitude affect our ability to assert ourselves in certain situations?

Take this opportunity to think of who you personally consider an 'authority figure', with yourself as the person needing help/assistance/guidance. People frequently find qualified professionals daunting figures. How would you feel if you found out that a client found you intimidating?

Of course the major drawback is that intimidated clients do not talk about what their problems are. They are likely to say they feel better, and everything is OK, because they don't want to be seen to cause a problem. One way to deal with this is to use 'immediacy'. Feed back to them what you feel the problem is.

It is important when communicating both verbally and by body language to avoid any patronising or 'parent' role. We all communicate in parent adult and child modes on a daily basis. However using any of the negative parent approaches is likely to elicit negative child responses, the main one being that of 'victim'. To communicate in an adult way is to use the full range of one's problem solving abilities. However there will be many times when a caring professional will need to assume a caring, rather than critical parent, role and it is the importance of knowing how to adapt your transactions to meet the immediate need that is important. If you have not already done so, you are recommended to read *Games People Play* by Eric Berne, the founder of Transactional Analysis, for more information on this subject.

A recent letter printed in a local newspaper was from a woman who was distressed and angry about Asians insisting on their own burial ground. This writer asked why they were not being cremated as she was aware that cremation was the practice in India. There are so many issues here, not least that she felt angry and helpless enough to have no other option than to write to the local press, but this sad ignorance of the vast difference between the cultural and religious practices of Moslems and Hindu people is quite widespread and representative, and we need to be constantly aware that our individual understanding is not necessarily shared throughout the community we work within or the people we work with. We need to consider, therefore, how much offence we can cause if we or colleagues display this sort of pitiful lack of understanding. Ignorance and racism are not necessarily the same thing; however ignorance can lead to behaviour that may be interpreted as racist and anyone attempting to work in the area of black and ethnic minority health care must acquaint themselves with essential information concerning religious and cultural aspects of care.

It is important not to assume, because a woman is wearing a sari, that she is necessarily Hindu or that a woman wearing a kameez and shalwar is always a Moslem. There are a considerable number of Christian Asians, for example, who may or may not wear the cultural dress adopted by Hindus and Moslems.

Listed below are a number of representative questions which anyone working with black and ethnic minorities should be able to answer.

- What are the five K's of Sikhism?
- What is Ramadan? The significance of Ramadan? Who may not be expected to comply, and under what circumstances?
- What is Diwali? How long does it last?

- What is a Hakim?
- What is the significance of the left and right hands for Moslems?
- Which culture may use root ginger to prevent travel sickness?
- Which culture may use a nutmeg in the mouth of stroke victims to encourage the regaining of muscle control?

The answers are not included so that you will be encouraged to find out the facts for yourself, some from earlier chapters of this book.

Another area of potential difficulty concerns English colloquial expressions. If you find yourself working in some parts of East London and a client says he or she is feeling 'Tom', you will need to know this means 'sick' ('Tom and Dick'). It is also wise to consider when talking with people whose first language is not English, that idiomatic phrases like 'under the weather', 'off colour', 'down in the mouth' or 'shaking like a leaf' may be confusing or totally misunderstood. (See also Chapter 9 for more information on communication.)

Alix Henley has written three very good basic reference works about Asian cultures, full details of which are given in the 'Further reading' section at the end of this book.

This chapter has concentrated on Asian people because in situations where there are both extreme cultural and language differences, communication difficulties and misunderstandings are most likely to arise. Difficulties may arise, however, within any interaction between people of differing cultures or people with differing backgrounds or ages from the same culture.

How can we better understand a culture? We can learn a lot from the written word, but so much more from direct participation and learning from people.

In her paper 'Ethnography: a tool for learning', Susan Dobson sets out a learning system that can be used by individuals or as a group project. Ethnography is a form of research that involves observation, participation, interviewing and interacting with people from the culture being learned about. It involves attending cultural functions of the group, observing activities and behaviour and recording a whole range of information.

Interviewing should be flexible and informal and, subject to the agreement of the interviewee, audiotapes might be made, life histories written down with perhaps a collection of relevant artifacts.

All these add up to a form of cultural discovery that no textbook will ever give you.

To do this, however, you do need an entry gate. It could be that you know a member of the group that you want to learn about. If not, a good method is to approach your local Community Relations Council with a clear explanation of your objective and your ultimate goal of being better able to provide/plan more sensitive services. If there is a group of you, each member of the group could investigate one culture with the results shared collectively at the end of the project. As your interest is particularly that of elderly people, this can be the focus for your study.

Irrespective of our individual cultural origins, we all pay our taxes which fund the Health and Social Services we receive. We therefore have a right to receive the support we need delivered sensitively by informed, caring professionals.

The Pre-Retirement Association has begun to address the issue of planning for retirement of ethnic minority groups, and has identified that, in addition to the issues of poverty, ageism, loneliness, and loss of esteem, there are additional issues to be addressed as the retired population consists of an increasing number of people from different cultures. These additional issues include cultural attitudes to retirement, racism, cultural requirements of food, hygiene and religion by statutory services, health needs, lack of knowledge of 'the system' for obtaining help, and communication – especially the language in which pre-retirement information is provided, which could then reach a wider audience. The programme planning should ideally be planned with consultation between employer, employees and representatives of local representative groups. The term PRE-retirement should not be overlooked.

Nothing is more effective than evidence of cultural understanding and an acceptance of a wide range of diversity among peoples. We are indeed fortunate to live in a multicultural and multi-linguistic society which, if we allow it, can only enrich all our lives.

To communicate these views to health and social service staff in a meaningful and effective way requires an experienced educator. All levels of the service need to be addressed, and the content will depend on local circumstances. A multicultural audience will not only focus the issues, but also ensure that cross cultural views are considered.

To gain an effective response, the importance of the issues must be emphasised, and practical examples and projects will produce the best results. The choice of presenter is also pertinent, and, from experience, the views of service users can be revealing and the most convincing message courier.

References

DOBSON, S. (1986). Ethnography: a tool for learning. *Nurse Education Today*, 6 (April): pp. 00–0.
ROGERS, C. (1942). *Counselling and Psychotherapy*. Houghton Mifflin, Boston.

21

Summary and recommendations

Amanda Squires

At the inception of the NHS in 1948, medical care was to be provided to all irrespective of race, religion or creed. The Race Relations Act (1976) acknowledged that Britain had become a multicultural society and the NHS and Community Care Act (1990) states that 'people from different cultural backgrounds may have particular care needs and problems'. Data on the population must be collected, plans made accordingly and myths verified.

Defining the population

The collection of such data may be sensitive, and must be collected in a way to ensure validity, community support and involvement and to enable the production of information to identify social and health needs. Interpretation of the data requires skill and an appreciation of the issues to be explored. The crude simplicity of many measures do not do justice to the complexities contained in the data. In detailed analysis of the elderly population, pensioner and sub-pensioner data should be examined so that planning of educational, occupational, communication, health and social needs can be addressed proactively and dynamically as the unprecedented population changes occur. Studies of take up of services will identify discrepancies – mainly due to lack of information or inappropriate presentation. Geographical distribution not only by city, but within that city is also very relevant: in certain areas the indigenous population may be a minority group. It should be noted that religious beliefs may be as significant as ethnicity, often determining food, alcohol and ritual requirements which need to be especially noted at times of ill health.

The history of migration will enable staff to put into context the issues described. Although Britain has never been an immigrant receiving country to the same extent as Australia or the United States, in 1981 6.3 per cent of the population were born outside the United Kingdom, with much local variation. The largest immigrant group is the Irish who, along with the Jewish, have for some time been significant minorities in the United Kingdom. Post war refugees from Europe were encouraged to migrate to assist with the labour shortage, as were later arrivals from Asia and the Caribbean. Although some immigrants have come with poor resources and seeking any employment, some have come with considerable skills and have become respected and wealthy businessmen and women.

Despite origins and reasons for migration, elderly people from minority groups facing old age will have the usual barriers to face such as prejudice and lack of access to services. When accompanied by communication difficulties, such problems may seem insurmountable.

Service planning in response to population profile

Having established a population profile, its local significance must be determined. An example is given of a pilot study to compare take up and identify presenting pathology in the majority and minority populations of a health district. Representatives of cultural groups should be invited to contribute to the data collection and interpretation process.

The voluntary sector supporting ethnic minority cultures is frequently hampered by lack of recognition, and lack of resources to gain recognition. Such services are essential for social support as well as acting as pressure groups to raise awareness, promote appropriate provision and facilitate communication with providers.

The departure from one's own country for a long period for what ever reason is emotional. When the reason for migration is the 'pull' factor, it can be stimulating but when it is the 'push' factor, such as persecution, it can be devastating. Even in the former as children grow up in the new culture, and grandchildren no longer speak the 'mother' tongue', isolation and depression can be very real. Interviews with elderly people from minority cultures ageing in another homeland reveal that loneliness is a major problem, and these factors should influence mental health, social and leisure provision.

Cultural concepts of health and disease are important issues. There are basically two models: Eastern (traditional) and Western and the beliefs, practices and expectations held must be appreciated. Elderly people, due to their illnesses being largely chronic and socially influenced, have special needs. The culture and conduct of the individual may influence his or her direction for seeking help and, increasingly, older people from minority groups are using traditional medicine in old age to address these chronic and social problems as they seek approachability, low cost, and ease of communication. These principles should be noted. For many a mix of styles of medicine may be practiced and consideration must be given to the wishes of patients to follow one, or both simultaneously. For an appreciation of the complementary or uncomplementary effects, and subsequent ethical considerations, knowledge is required.

Morbidity for some conditions is high in minority groups but is balanced by lower morbidity in other conditions giving a similar total mortality rate in comparison with the indigenous population. In general, initial migrants tend to be fitter than those who stay behind or who followed to join families, but the 'healthy migrant' effect tends to wear off and the health profile of the country of origin is adopted. The main differences are respiratory disease and related psychiatric problems in the Irish, coronary heart disease and diabetes in South Asians, and strokes and diabetes in Afro-Caribbeans. The differences must be noted and plans made accordingly with appropriate staff education.

The needs of ethnic minority elders in many areas are not yet known – and their unrepresentative numbers of users probably reflects lack of knowledge of access. A colour-blind service may appear to offer 'equality' but, where take up is disproportionate, questions must be asked of appropriateness, awareness, access and acceptability.

Managers will need to plan their service and education of staff as an ongoing commitment. Policies need to include the needs of ethnic minorities as central – not as an afterthought – with monitoring of the results. One-off limited projects can be seen as token commitment. Recruitment of staff from minority groups will not only assist in the education of colleagues and ensure appropriate provision and information, but will reflect commitment to equal opportunity. Education of staff at all levels is essential, and input from elders themselves will focus the subject and dispel myths and stereotypes. Training on issues relating to race should be an on-going part of the staff educational programme. Staff who undertake their tasks in the client's own home will gain more cultural awareness, and will need responsive social skills.

Service delivery

Having established the population profile and its resulting health and social needs, the next step is to ensure that relevant staff groups are aware of the composition and significance of their population to enable them to provide services, and that information on those services is available to all sections of the population via appropriate media. The additional time needed for these activities should be noted.

Education of clients as to the purpose of the provision of equipment, drugs, activities and other procedures will need explanation in advance of treatment provision; lack of information is the most common cause of complaint. Public relations exercises can be promoted through the various organisations – but will have to be in appropriate language and media. Illiteracy in the mother tongue and use of video is often underestimated in minority groups.

The quality of the first contact with the service is essential, and the method of communication should be well planned. Assessment of need by the appropriate worker is key, and must be comprehensive with the client feeling part of the decision making process. General information on the culture of the client will have been established, but individuality must be central. Although practical help is often emphasised, counselling often has an enhanced role with minority groups and may fall to any team member who should be prepared in advance by an appreciation of the issues. To ensure wider needs are met, liaison between services is essential. Outpatient and day care, and even more so inpatient and residential care provision, must ensure that attitudes – not only between staff and clients but also between clients – are conducive to the purpose of that service provision.

Those currently providing high quality services for elderly people should have no difficulty in incorporating the needs of elderly people from ethnic minority groups, as the ingredients of provision based on knowledge, staff attitudes, education and planning will be continually addressed.

It is no longer possible to manage health care resources without consideration and planning for the management of ethnic minority elders.

Recommendations

1. Data base

A local population data base of ethnic structure, health needs and service take up is needed.

2. Local resource

Elders from minority groups have the knowledge that is being sought and should be encouraged to share it.

The training of carers is essential to complement service provision.

Voluntary groups representing or including the needs of ethnic minority elders should be encouraged and their work made known especially to community based staff.

3. Service provision

Morbidity and mortality of different groups must be appreciated and plans made accordingly for prevention and treatment.

Appropriate leisure activities are an important component of health and social care.

4. Communication

Communication is a prerequisite for appropriate care and can be by a variety of means.

The appearance of staff, buildings and directions should encourage approachability.

5. Information

The roles of different providers should be explained so that access and expectations are understood.

Pre-retirement courses should include the health needs of minority groups.

6. Education

Education of all staff at all levels in transcultural medicine is essential.

7. Research

Research on service provision and outcomes should be on-going and the results fed back for appropriate action.

Traditional medical practices should be understood and incorporated or complemented where appropriate and contraindications noted.

Useful addresses

Age Concern (England)
Astral House
1268 London Road
London SW16 4EJ
Tel: 081-679 8000

Age Exchange Theatre Trust
Age Exchange Reminiscence Centre
11 Blackheath Village
London SE3 9LA
Tel: 071-318 9105/3504

British Geriatric Society
1 St Andrews Place
Regents Park
London NW1
Tel: 071-935 4004

British Red Cross Society (Multi ethnic affairs dept)
3 Grosvenor Crescent
London SW1X 7ES
Tel: 071-235 3241

CHOICE magazine
Bedford Chambers
Covent Gardens
London WC2E 8HA

Commission for Racial Equality
Elliot House
10–12 Allington Street
London SW1E 5EH
Tel: 071-828 7022

Diploma in Geriatric Medicine
The Royal College of Physicians
11 St Andrew Place
London NW1 4LE
Tel: 071-935 1174

EXTEND (Exercise training for the elderly and/or disabled)
1a North Street
Sherringham
Norfolk NR26 8LJ

Help The Aged
St James Walk
London EC1R 0BE
Tel: 071-253 0253

National Extension College
1 Brooklands Avenue
Cambridge
CB2 2HN

Pre-Retirement Association
Nodus Centre
University of Surrey Campus
Guildford
Surrey GU2 5RX
Tel 0483 39323

Research Institute for Care of the Elderly
St Martin's Hospital
Coombe Down.
Bath
Tel 0225 835866

Sickle Cell Society
Green Lodge
Barretts Green Road
London NW10
Tel: 081-961 7795/4006/8346

SAGA Holidays
Folkestone
Kent

Thalassaemia Society United Kingdom
107 Nightingale Lane
London N8
Tel 081-348-0437/2553

Walthamstow Asian Elderly Concern
c/o Leyton Baths
Leyton High Road
Leyton
London E10

Further reading and resources

Books

Cruikshank, J. K. and Reevers, D. G. (1989). *Ethnic Factors in Health and Disease*, John Wright, London.

Fru, F. and Glendenning, F. (1989). *Black and Ethnic Minority Elders: Retirement Issues*. Pre-Retirement Association of Great Britain and Northern Ireland, London.

Henley, A. (1983) *Asians in Britain. Vol 1: Caring for Sikhs and their Families – Religious Aspect of Care. Vol 2: Caring for Muslims and their Families – Religious Aspects of Care. Vol 3: Caring for Hindus and their Families – Religious Aspects of Care.* Health Education Council and National Extension College, Cambridge.

Mares, P., Henley, A. and Baxter, C. (1985) *Health Care in Multiracial Britain.* Health Education Council and National Extension College, Cambridge.

McAvoy, B. R. and Donaldson, L. (1990) *Health Care for Asians*. Oxford Medical Publications, Oxford.

Neuberger, J. (1987). *Caring for Dying People of Different Faiths*. Austen Cornish, London.

Qureshi, B. (1989). *Transcultural Medicine: Dealing with Patients from Different Cultures*. Kluwer Academic Publishers, Lancaster.

Thompson, M. K. (1990). *Commonsense Geriatrics*. Clinical Press, Bristol.

The Forgotten People: A Book on Carers in Three Minority Ethnic Communities in Southwark. Available from Bailey Distribution, Dept. D/KFP, Warner House, Folkestone, Kent CT19 6PH.

Training packs and videos

Henley, A. *Asian Foods and Diets*. (Training pack and slides). Available from National Extension College, Cambridge.

Afro-Caribbean Foods and Diets. (Training pack and slides). Available from 229 Woodhouse Lane, Leeds L52 9LF.

Chinese Foods and Diets. (Training pack and slides). Available from 229 Woodhouse Lane, Leeds.

A Taste of Health. (Video on general nutrition for Asians). Available from 229 Woodhouse Lane, Leeds.

Asian Carers. (A video and booklet for Asian Carers in Leicester). Available from Voluntary Action Leicester, 32 De Montfort Street, Leicester LE1 7GD.

According to Need: Services Available for Older People in a Multiracial Society. (Video). Available from Age Concern (England).